Walking Away

Waking up from the American Dream

MICHELE MAINGOT CABRAL

2-13-15

To Sagen & Kent,
Our favorite fellow
travelers! Can't
wait to explore
together and play
in the mud!
Love,
Michele + Mike

This book is dedicated to my parents and their parents from whom I inherited the ability to always land on my feet. It is a helpful quality since they also passed on the "adventure gene" which impels me to consistently jump from high places. It is also dedicated to my husband Mike who is always ready in case I fall.

CONTENTS

AKNOWLEDGMENTS

I would like to extend special thanks to my readers and mentors: Theresa Small Sneed, Kathy Doore, Lee Goggin, and Kent Black. Thank you also to Johnny Craik for the cover photograph. Thank you to my teachers, both the decided and the inadvertent. Thank you to my family for understanding my need to do this and to Mike who has taught me to embrace my imperfections.

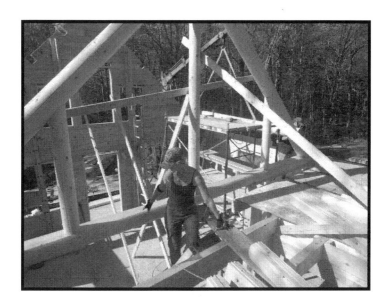

PROLOGUE
April 12, 2014

"Honey, I want you to bring your little desk with you next time you drive down to see us. I have such wonderful memories of you as a little girl sitting at that desk writing your poetry." It was a familiar sentiment from my mom who still has my bridesmaid dress from my cousin's wedding in the 1980's.

"I know Mom, but I don't have room for anything that serves no real purpose other than for sentimental reasons. If I store it in the basement, it will get ruined. It is time for some other little girl to sit at that desk and dream of being a writer someday. I am going to trade it in for a cool piece of furniture for the bathroom sink. I know you'll like it."

"You've had that desk since you were five and it has gone with you everywhere you have gone. It's your little poet's desk."

"So true, Mom. It has always reminded me of my

greater purpose in life. I have carried it around like a big talisman. Now it is time for me to finally be that writer. And poets must travel light. Besides it's the memory that counts and memories are very light."

"I guess you're right."

"Thanks Mom, I knew you'd understand. You have always been my biggest fan. It is time for your little poet to finally realize her dream."

That morning I cleared out years of assorted papers, stationary, letters, pictures, old passports, fountain pens, cute little erasers, rusty paperclips, third-grade report cards, and weird souvenirs of my life's journey. I was getting the desk ready for its trade. I paused on one bundle of papers. It was ten years of pink slips I had received from my school department in Rhode Island along with the rescind notices.

No wonder I had felt fatigued by my job. Every Valentine's Day for the past ten years I have gone through the emotional upheaval of not knowing if I would be employed the following year. It takes the steam right out of you but you have to keep up the same happy, excited face every day at work or the kids will crush you and make you miserable. It takes a lot of energy to keep up the game. While I was teaching English I didn't care because the literature fed me. However, because of budget cuts, I had to apply for a more bureaucratic position, and the game became harder to play.

There it was, in a little bundle of envelopes shoved into the desk drawer, all of the reasons that Mike and I decided to move off the grid, to simplify, and begin a new American Dream for ourselves. It was time, we decided, that we honor our lives' purposes. His, he claims, is to serve me. It sounds unlikely, but it is what he constantly tells me. I know differently; he was meant to invent better ways to do things and share that gift with other people. Mike is a modern day Ben Franklin (sometimes the genius, sometimes the turkey). We both have a dream of untethering our natural sense of creativity and adventure, to allow it to be the guiding force in our lives.

When the two of us paddled our kayaks up the Allagash Waterway in Northern Maine some years ago, we made a commitment to awaken from the American Dream which had become a nightmare for us of high numbers and low gain. The stress of keeping the dream going was killing us quietly. Our goal from that summer forward was to construct our own dream, a dream that would free us to honor our own cycles and rhythms. It would be something that would allow us to align with our creative natures, no matter how contrary to the mainstream current it would be.

As these thoughts circled around my head the day of the desk-clearing, I happened upon a little silver band that fit perfectly around my right ring finger. It reminded me of a commitment. It was inscribed with one simple word.

The word is *dream.*

It is time.

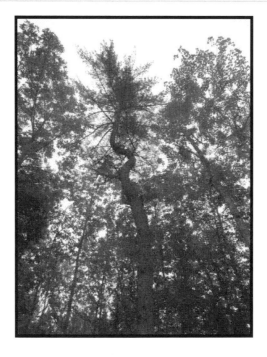

1. BEING MINDFUL
June 29, 2013

It's not so much the sound as it is the smell of a two-stroke engine that seeps into the recesses of my childhood memories and makes me think of the summer I discovered self-empowerment.

Memory takes me back to the day I experienced the thrill of waterskiing with friends and the first time I slalomed. I remember pushing all of my weight forward into my right leg to allow my left leg to fly free in the air and then let it land neatly in its nest behind my right leg. I had never considered myself very athletic but that day I experienced how listening to advice, processing it through my brain, and being mindful of my own body could make the impossible happen.

Today my husband Mike and I have had to dominate the impossible. We are following a shared dream of building a house "way up there" in the Maine woods with our own two hands. Our plan is to have no mortgage payments and only one house bill (taxes) - a pipe dream to some. Like every other impossible task anyone has ever done, we went about it systematically. We saved every penny we could and searched until we found our sacred piece of property on a beautiful river that sings all year long. We began our journey step-by-step.

With images of the Lorax circulating through our brains, we made a pact that we would always be mindful stewards of our land. We were thrilled that we would only have to cut down a few trees since the previous owner had already cleared the land for a house. I didn't want to touch a single tree, except to hug it and protect it from any harm.

Seven years later, after saving, planning, raising the kids, and learning about living off the grid, we were finally ready to build our little log cabin by the river. However, in the process of obtaining our building permits, we discovered that the site the previous owner had cleared was 100 feet too close to the river. The town's code officer marked out a new spot, way back in the woods where I was sure I would never get a view of the river, even from the loft window.

Mike, in his inimitable way, pointed out the irony of the environmentalists and their regulations that would force us to cut down at least a half an acre of trees instead of use the spot already cleared. Being an eternal optimist and not willing to let a bad attitude get in the way of our dream, he also pointed out that we would still be able to hear the river from our new spot. With a little judicious pruning here and there, he reasoned, we would have a beautiful view anyway. Also, being lovers of natural places, we both appreciate that building is regulated to protect the wilderness.

So with the little home-owner-sized chainsaw we were using for our property in Rhode Island, we began to clear our spot in the woods. My husband had helped other people cut down trees but was not well-practiced. Being a city girl, I had never wielded an axe. Before we began to cut the first tree, we discussed our strategy. I would find a spot out of the way and would tell him when and in which direction the tree would fall. Like all new things we decide to do together, we approached it from a cerebral perspective first. He thought about angles, researched it on line, and then lined up the smaller trees with definite leanings first, leaving the more difficult trees to cut last.

After the first tree landed, the nasty red hives that show up on Mike's temples calmed down and a visible confidence began to set into him. We still remained reverent for the power of the trees and reminded each other to be mindful as we worked.

It took us half a day just to fell our first little tree, process it into eighteen-inch segments for the wood pile, load the chunks into a wheel barrow that kept getting caught up on little stumps and valleys in the terrain, and drag out the branches to a spot away from the house. We had approximately seventy sizeable trees to cut down and a lot of brushy stuff to clear. Since we were both still working in Rhode Island, we had only three long weekends to get it all done. We had to hurry and take our time. More than a few trees looked impossible, like an eighty-foot white pine with a cork-screwed shape that could fall in any direction.

As we surveyed the land with the town inspector, he looked up at the towering giant and said, "Yep, you'll have to be very careful with that one. Could be a right widow-maker if you don't know what you're doing."

We thought about asking someone else to do it for us but had not factored the expense into our budget. We had counted on the already cleared lot in our careful planning. No time for despair.

We considered asking our nephew (an arborist) to drive up and help with his larger, better equipment but we would naturally have to pay him and it would cost us less money to just invest in our own. That's when we decided to purchase the top-of-the-line chainsaw (The Husky) that we take care of like a pet. After a little internet research, we invested in a large

(1200 pound capacity) Gorilla Cart with four wheels and suspension that made stacking our wood much more efficient. These are tools, we discussed, that we will use for many years to come since we will be heating and cooking with wood most of the year.

Armed with my two friends, Cindy (a pair of huge loppers) and Molly (a good little hatchet), I was able to process the tops of the trees, dragging them to spots along our driveway so that we can chip them later for mulch in our garden. Needless to say, I have gotten pretty good with an axe. As my husband reminds me, I must be mindful of the follow through and always watch to keep my fingers and limbs out of the way of the arc.

And so, between driving back and forth to finish up work in Rhode Island and sell the family home, we have been able to clear our lot and create quite a sizeable wood pile. We also have learned that while Dr. Seuss was right about cutting trees and paving over natural habitats, the trees are okay with our work.

All except Old Corker, the eighty foot white pine. It kicked my husband's backside and sent him flying. This happened after the tree was already on the ground and we were chopping it up. That was the moment that we were extremely glad that we bought the better chain saw since it has a number of safety features. Old Corker earned our respect that day and we will think of its gravitas every time we load it into our wood stove.

We have honored the energy of our trees by processing them down to logs that are two-inch in diameter, even the pine trees since we bought a wood stove with a powerful catalytic burn. We also have learned the difference, not just in leaves and bark, but weight and power between a beech and a birch. I will know what to feed the stove for a quick burn or for an all-nighter. "If you want to keep warm while you sleep, head for the beech…" we sing while we stack the iron-heavy segments.

I know how sweet a freshly-fallen beech smells when you cut it. I know what the heart-wood of a maple looks like and have marveled at the sometimes bright orange inner bark of a birch. I know that a tree definitely makes a sound when it falls in the woods, even if no human is around to hear it. If it's an eighty-foot white pine with an especially bad attitude, it cracks, wheezes, and reverberates as it booms to the ground.

My city-girl legs and arms have deep scratches and black-fly bites all over them. I smile as I look at my activity badges since they remind me of the summer legs I always had as a kid. I am sure that I will have little scars here and there for a while. They probably won't last as long as all of the wood we have stockpiled.

I have learned to drag out the branches of the white and red oaks to particular spots in the woods since they are seeding right now and will plant more oaks than ever before. Nature will take its course and the forest around us will be more robust than ever with all of the new movement.

Through friends, we learned about the wonders of the white pine pollen and have gathered it from Old Corker to give to them to make some tinctures. We have felt the cool, pink flesh of the white pine and tasted it in memory of Yule Gibbons (not so bad). We have made tea from its leaves (pretty good).

After clearing our lot, I am getting excited about planting some fruit trees near the house and allowing the maples to grow in while keeping the little scratchy hemlocks at bay. Clearing our lot allows the maples and oaks to grow stronger and healthier. We decided that this fall will be good for collecting acorns, judging by the number already on the trees we felled. We can't wait to make our own flour blends and top off our confections with our homemade maple syrup.

We are also getting excited about using the original lot that was cleared seven years ago by the previous owner. Our plan for raised beds and moveable chicken coop will work wonderfully there. We map out the wild rabbit-eyed blueberry bushes all over the property and the wild blackberry growing in patches all throughout the previously cleared lot since they get plenty of sun. We remark to each other how happy our bees will be here when we finally can move them up. It will all work out just fine my husband tells me.

There is just one small problem: the garden plots now

must be cleared for our raised beds. It won't take the Husky chainsaw but will take several days with Cindy Loppers and Molly Hatchet to get it ready. Seven years after the previous owner had cleared the plot for his house, nature has reclaimed her own. She has replanted the forest and I have to report, it is doing famously!

And so, being mindful stewards of our land takes on a new meaning. It means respecting the fact that we are part of the land now. It means that as mindful stewards, we must realize that everything gives and it is better to both give and receive.

The smell of a two-stroke engine also takes on new meaning this summer. It smells of the way that my husband and I depend on each other, not just to look out for the trajectory of an eighty-foot pine tree as it thuds to the ground or to research better equipment and budget for it. The two-stroke reminds me of the way we depend on one another to be mindful: to hydrate, stop when we are tired, watch out for the arc of a hatchet swing, laugh and make up songs while we labor, to take pictures, to make construction cookies, and to pause every now and then to eat them.

The smell of the chain saw reminds me that it is empowering to challenge what we previously considered to be impossible. It is a reminder that what we might not possess in natural ability and experience, we can always make up for by heeding good advice and being mindful: two important features of a good brain.

THINGS THAT MADE THE CUT
(We are glad we kept or bought)

Most of these items will be mentioned in subsequent chapters but it bears attention here in list form.

* A really big chain saw: 20" Husky, gorilla cart, and 33 ton log splitter
* Garden tools: Loppers and clippers, axes, hatchets, shovels, come along, etc.
* The Conservo steam oven and a hand-operated grain mill
* Cast iron pans, including a cool bread pan that makes 12 little bread loafs
* Large pressure cooker for canning, food dehydrator, hand-cranked pasta maker
* Construction tools including biscuit joiner, routers and forstner bits
* Bulk oils, essential oils, and equipment for making salves, lip balm, and soap
* All books on wildflowers, edible wild plants, trees, birds, gardening, house building
* Radios and music playing devices
* Assorted lamps, electric and propane
* Stainless steel pots, especially the two gallon pot for canning and cheese-making
* Toys, puzzles, kaleidoscopes, kites, sporting equipment
* Fabric, sewing machine, and crafting materials (came in handy during Christmas)
* Wool blankets, sweaters, outerwear, and socks (and all wool yarn)
* *A very special little desk that I have owned since I was a kid*

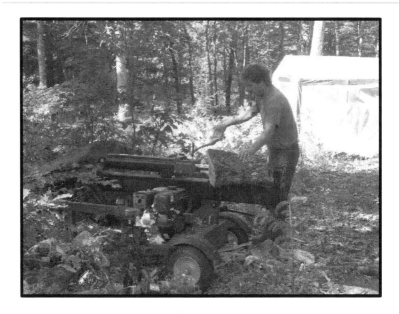

2. LESSONS FROM TREES
July 14, 2013

While Mike and I build our log cabin way out here in the woods, we get a few visitors/ helpers who camp with us. I often think that once we build the house, I hope we continue to camp out with our friends because sleeping outside under the trees gives me a renewed perspective on who I am and who I want to be.

As a mother of two girls in their early twenties, I have a tendency to worry about them. The ins and outs of their lives preoccupies me. However, I have recently come to realize, as I worry about them, other family members, and my friends, that good relationships are better served when I am like the trees under which I place my tent.

The trees look on and are readily available to provide us shade and comfort if we seek it from them. They watch as we go about our lives, most times ignored by us, but never involving themselves in our business. In short, they are here for us but are completely free to go about their own business while leaving us to mind our own.

The trees on our property will provide us with a buffer from the Northern winds of winter, fuel our wood stove to keep us warm and fed, have kept us cool in the summer, deliver us with the logs and lumber for our outbuildings, serve a complex ecosystem for other flora and fauna, and offer a connection to the earth for humans that is best felt, not described.

The trees have provided me with a certain wisdom that has been an integral part of the process I am going through as I shift from the industrial grid to the natural grid of life in the woods. Some of the things my husband and I have had to change have not been easy. Things like getting rid of our crock pot or adjusting to using an outhouse while we build our house are easy compared to the emotional adjustments I have had to make.

Being off the grid makes me worry about a few things that mothers worry about. My cell phone is not the most reliable out here because of the heavy tree cover. I have to go into town to get internet access for e-mail, Facebook, and immediate news coverage. (What if another horrible occurrence happens in their city?) I worry that my daughters can't get to me easily by train or bus, and well, the list goes on but you get the idea. There is plenty to worry about. Then add to that our parents and friends who might need us and my list of worries continues.

Our cell phone culture has created a circumstance where if someone can't reach you after a few tries, they get frustrated and worried. I know, it happens to me all of the time with my own daughters.

Yet, I think back to when we were in our twenties. We got ourselves into plenty of stuff that either taught us a good lesson or changed the course of our lives, but either way, it was our own business, and we had to take care of it ourselves. We never expected our parents (or anyone else for that matter) to solve our problems for us. Like the trees, they were there to provide a little temporary shelter and comfort if we needed it, but we would have to seek it from them. Otherwise, they would just go about their lives until such time. There was no mechanism to hover over us and scrutinize every detail of how we were living. They had to look at the bigger picture.

So, I sit under the trees and I think, this is how I need to be. I need to feel free to just mind my own business. I need to feel comfortable with the fact that, like the trees, I will go largely ignored by my kids until they need a little comfort and have reached a time when they will stop and are silent in my presence. Perhaps it is the silence of the trees that helps us find wisdom, perhaps it is the slow steady growth, the reaching upward, or the tree energy that is equally of heaven and earth, the way that we are.

Our "reach out and touch someone" culture has created unnecessary anxiety. Due to social media, we are so connected presently that we can follow every life's detail of our friends and loved ones. They are captured in snapshots that are sometimes misleading. I look at pictures of my cousins on the beach and I think, "Wow, they look so much happier than I am." If I stop to think about it for a moment, I would realize that we spend a lifetime practicing a smile for the camera. Back before the snapshot, when photographs were rare, people never smiled for the camera. Were they any less happy? Is the prospect of happiness just a false promise like prospecting for gold where none is ever found?

My father once told me that feeling happy is perhaps less important than feeling content. I ruminate on this idea as I shift into a completely new arena of daily living. I think to myself, "yes, I no longer draw a paycheck, am expected anywhere, have to get up and place a smile on my face, but I am still working. My adult daughters no longer really need me the way they did when they were kids." My sense of happiness is a little uprooted as I am experiencing a strange gap where the feeling of being needed used to ground me.

Of course I am still needed. Just as humans need the trees. But we don't need them too close to the house because they will cause a liability. We need them as a framework for our lives, just as our friends and families need each other, as a framework. We need to provide comfort when asked, but for the most part, we need to be free to go about our own business.

Like the trees under which I camp, it is good for my daughters to go about their lives unencumbered by me and my judgments. My parents and friends would rather I be content than a bundle of worry. Of this, I am absolutely sure, just as I would rather that my own daughters feel at peace with their lives. I do not want them to worry about me out here under the cover of trees, a little less accessible than I would be in a town, getting paid in eggs and Swiss chard.

What they do need from me is a sense of calm, a feeling that being content in life is possible. Mostly they need my silence, my neutral presence that provides a framework for their own lives. They need to be able to seek me and find someone who is still actively growing, stretching upward while staying grounded.

I am a natural-born tree hugger. I need to touch their power and hold it close to my heart. Just like the trees, I am best to just watch and wait in a calm, neutral position, allowing all to be happy when they seek my company. Trees require nothing of me, not even a sense that I will be gentle with them. They wait and listen, hoping that my sounds will be beautiful and lyrical. They bend and reach, true, but movement was not built into their prototypes. The most a tree will ever fly is when it is in seed form.

Yet, trees know that eventually all life will come to them, even if it is when they fall, their final movement.

STAYING CONNECTED

After a year of being able to only text message from our house and of calls being dropped from the "phone booth" on our front deck, we devised a plan.

Mike was sure that the only way to make calls was to stand on the deck, raise his hands in the air and proclaim to the world, "I am the All-Powerful Orb!!!!" It usually worked.

We finally acquired a cell phone booster (use the made in America one, it is the only one that really works well). Mike attached it the roof of the house. We attached it to a surge protector so that we can turn it off when we don't need it to save solar power. Now we don't lose our calls and can use our phones for internet access. We prefer the pay-as-you-go variety since contracts just bug us. By shutting off our solar inverter at night, we can disable the whole system so we don't sleep with unnecessary electro-magnetic waves running through us.

We tried using our phones as a wireless hotspot but decided the extra charges weren't worth it. I have been saving my files to a cloud and e-mailing them to myself when I am in town so that if I need to email from my phone, I can just access the files from the cloud or my e-mail.

Our friends visit us, expecting it to be like "Little House on the Prairie." Truth is, we are employing the latest in technology in our house. Sometimes we just shut down the booster so they can disconnect while they're here. It's kind of a subtle meddling but is entirely benevolent.

Every day the world gets less and less wired. We want them to be also.

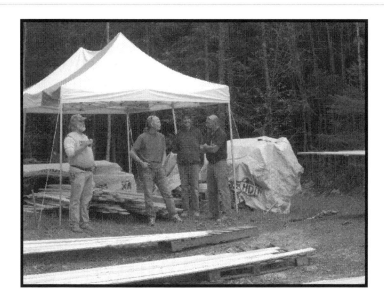

3. LIFE WITHOUT A JOB
September 23, 2013

Adjusting to an off-the-grid lifestyle has its merits. It leaves room for spontaneity in life. Yesterday, instead of spending most of my day cooped up in a classroom of adolescents, I was outside collecting and processing acorns, marveling at the bounties of nature.

I walked through the woods with my dog Hermes by my side, sat by the river and crushed some acorns with a stone in an old potato bag. I tied a knot in the bag and attached a rope to it, walked down to the river and found a good spot for leaching them. I guessed that in a few days I would go back and see if they taste bland. If not, I will leave them in a little longer.

As I worked, the sun sparkled on the water and the sound of the river bathed me in peace. Becoming aware of the sound of the wind and the harmony it plays with the river, my thoughts were light and floated downstream.

Heading back up to camp, I stopped and collected more

acorns. The oak trees have been dropping their acorns for more than a month and they land with such force that they pop and cause Hermes to growl. We joke about his being startled by acorns but they sound pretty forceful. Even though we are using every last resource and bit of energy to get our house finished and weather-tight for the winter, we still know that we can't pass up gathering the acorns right now. They are just so fat and juicy this year that the next few years could be pretty slim pickings. Nature has her cycles. We knew we would regret it later if we didn't gather as many as we could right away before the bugs get to them.

Mike was busy with shingling the roof of the house, no easy task on a 12/12 pitch and all alone. Way up there, it was helpful to have a ground crew available. I had been torn, should I stay around the house while he worked, busying myself with little organizational jobs that make the construction site less stressful in many ways, waiting to start the generator for him pick up a tool he dropped, pass up supplies, or should I gather acorns?

His answer was, "Well, we will be sorry we didn't when the snow falls and they are all covered." He descended from the roof, grabbed his gathering bucket, and joined me. We love working together, no matter the task, but we especially love foraging together. It is a singular pleasure we share.

Within a half an hour, a couple of friends arrived to offer some help with the house. They saw us with our buckets and grabbed theirs. We walked down to the river, skidded on slippery leaves and laughed. I showed them my leeching experiment and we discussed different methods. Being herbalists and naturalists, they showed me mare's tail, wild rose, a type of wild mint, winter berry, and another creeper with blue, dusty berries we took back to camp to look up. On the way, we stopped to collect more acorns, marveling at the size and weight of the kernels.

We talked about how nature seems to provide more for us when we are willing to stop and appreciate her beauty and generosity. When we honor her gifts, we discover she offers us so much more. By simply bending down and seeing the world from a closer vantage point, for instance, we find more berries on a blueberry bush that are larger and sweeter than any others we found before. We discussed plants and their interactions with us if we stop to listen. We shared thoughts about medicinal properties, Shakespeare, and little discoveries.

Digging through the accumulating layers of fallen leaves, I found a tiny collection of small yellow and peach colored orbs.

"Hey, I wonder what this is?"

"It looks like a little storage shed for a mouse or chipmunk. Those are seeds," my friend Heather answered.

"Wow, I thought they might be spores or something." I quickly covered it up, trying not to disturb our tiny friend's home. Whoever it was had been working hard to store up for the winter, the same way I was. I appreciated its work and planning. I silently said a reverent word for its well-being and prosperity.

Glenn chimed in. "It reminds me of the hunting story one of the elders from our gathering told about feeding the squirrels and chipmunks when he hunted so that he became their friends and they wouldn't reveal his location in the woods. They would climb all over him."

I might have to try that, I thought. Hunting deer isn't that easy.

Gathering with friends in our new work world means connecting on many levels and sharing. It means room for spontaneity and shared joys. It had been drizzling most of the afternoon but the rain intensified. We all ducked under the canopy of our camper and I made some herbal tea and popcorn on the camp stove. We were happy to stay dry and warm but remarked at how much time most people normally spend indoors. I thought about how I had spent the entire day outside, adding or subtracting layers of wool and down as needed.

"I am hardening off," I said to Heather. It is best to get the body used to the cold in natural increments to give it time to adjust. We do it for our plants, why not for our bodies? We laughed at the truth of it and discussed how in the working world we would already be surrounded by a controlled environment of hot air all day long.

"It's stifling," she said.

There are a lot of things that are stifling about the working world. I guess that's why I am willing to have nothing in order to be free of it. Don't get me wrong. I think you would be hard-pressed to find anyone who has worked as hard as I have in the last six months. Building a house is a major undertaking. A husband and wife team that is building 90% of it on their own with a limited budget is quite another thing. Add to that the fact that we have done most of it working from a camper with no refrigerator, heat, or running water, you're talking a lot of little jobs most people don't have to do such as cart water from the river or pump rain water into the camper to wash dishes in a sink. I would say, not working has been plenty of work.

When my best friend visits us to help us build our house, she marvels at the way that Mike and I have not only been building at a record pace, but have also foraged and set aside a lot of food for the winter. We have canned and set aside blueberry, blackberry, and autumn olive jam, hot pickled milkweed pods, and hard apple cider, as well as various cordials and a few herbal infusions. We have dried herbs for teas and stored walnuts.

We are now processing the acorns and will be canning up some pumpkins I got from our local farmer down the road for a reduced price. I have used the walnut hulls to dye some tired or ugly wool sweaters that we picked up second hand and have refurbished some of our wardrobe.

It has been fun to see what I can recycle. One success was a pair of my husband's light khaki work pants that I just could not get to look clean with all of the glues and grout stains from his work. I popped them right into the bucket of dye and they look pretty good now.

Don't try this using an old pair of rubber gloves, though. Mine were worn and my thumbs still have a brown hue to them. It's the kind of stain you have to simply grow out of. Good thing I don't have to show up at work with these hands! I can just picture how I would have to hide them under the table at our meetings or devise ways to avoid using the chalk board for a few weeks.

Yesterday I took a morning walk down to the river to refresh my memory of Heather's plant lessons and my thoughts drift. I think about how much I am learning and growing out here. I think about how strong I have gotten when most people my age are becoming frail.

Mike still runs into town a few times a month to do an odd flooring job here and there because we do need money for food staples, gas, propane, snow tires, and all of the odds and ends that building a house requires. My job, I tell myself, is to do what I can without money. And to write. I think I am earning my keep.

ANY-BERRY DELIGHTS

We happen to have a lot of low-laying blueberry bushes on our property. They are sweet and profuse. This year we gathered a good supply of wild blueberries, blackberries, and our favorite: autumn olive berries.

Autumn olive is a wild invasive that grows all over New England. I wouldn't be surprised if it has drifted north and south along the highways. Once you know what it is, you'll start to see it everywhere. Most New Englanders consider it an obstinate pest but we absolutely love the plant. First of all, the berries are positively delicious. Secondly, they are gorgeously abundant; one or two plants will yield enough for a five gallon bucket. Thirdly, they are an amazing super food that the Chinese have treasured for eons.

If you follow the healthful benefits of fruits and vegetables and know what phytochemicals and lycopene are, you will appreciate this statistic from Cornell: autumn olive berries contain seventeen times the amount of lycopene as a tomato. I'm sure you're impressed. When you consider how willingly these plants produce without any human intervention and compare it to what it takes to cultivate a tomato, well, you can see why we like them so much.

So, what do you do with them once you find them? Wash them, cook them for 20 minutes, mash them in a food mill, add a small amount of sugar, and can them for a jam that even jam-haters will like. (You can get the full recipe on-line easily.)

Our favorite method is to make fruit leather from it: cook with no water, add very little sugar, and pour a thickened liquid onto yoghurt container lids that we place on the racks of our dehydrator. You can buy special plastic trays for making fruit leathers for your dehydrator but we use the plastic container tops and they work very well. Stack with wax paper.

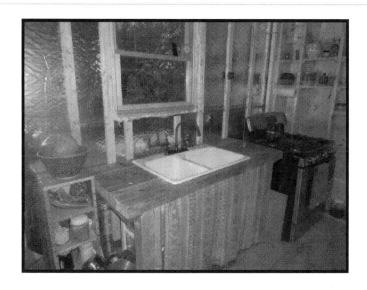

4. IT TAKES TWO
October 13, 2013

I am watching the sun set from the windows of our new house as the river peeks through the trees with a steel blue glint. The waxing moon dominates a fading blue sky while the bright little light of Venus smiles through a pink swath of horizon. I marvel at nature's beauty while I wait for my husband to come home from a day at work. It was an emergency call: someone started a job but couldn't finish it. His original plan for the day had been to get started on the front steps to the house since we have been using ladders and ramps to get to the deck. We had our first snow a few days ago and I fell off the icy ladder. That morning it became apparent that we had better get going on the stairs to the front porch.

With winter well on its way, there are quite a few things we had better get to. The only problem is that there are only two of us and we need money to buy the materials for what is left. So when Matt from the store called and asked Mike if he could hurry over and finish a tile job, he had no choice but to say yes, he'd be over in an hour.

Left alone, I decided to sand down the kitchen countertop Mike made out of packing lumber. He used a biscuit joiner and wood glue to create a butcher block countertop for me. I also moved some of our clothes over to the house from the camper, made a pot of Boston baked beans on the wood stove, and moved a cord of firewood over from the front of the house to the back where we will build the woodshed next spring. I was busy and happy.

Driven back into the house from the cold and the fading light, Hermes accompanied me as I warmed up by the fire. Other than the light from my computer as I write this, the only light around me is from the woodstove and a small candle. I can't wait for Mike to come home to add some light to my world as he always does. I expect he will bounce up the construction plank with a huge smile and say how glad he is to be home. He will mention that something smells really good and tell me how much he loves me.

While building our house, I have discovered how strong and able I can be. I have also discovered how much I need Mike. The truth is, we need each other. Living out here on the edge is a little different than living close to a large number of people. Out here, we really do need each other. He needs to know that while he is out working for money, I am at home making sure things are in order. He needs to know he will come home to a warm house, some dinner, and a friend. It sounds a little old fashioned but it works.

As I meet more and more couples who live self-sufficient lifestyles, I recognize a certain bond that they share. I get a sense that their relationship is based on strong mutual respect. I may be wrong, but my sense is that they would no sooner betray their partner than cut off an arm, since the results could lead to similar hardships. These are people who absolutely need one another to survive. Living this lifestyle would be nearly impossible alone, though I am sure some do it.

It takes two to cut and stack enough wood for the winter, gather and process wild foods, plan and budget for necessary tools and materials, build, till, plant, and harvest, feed everyone, and maintain everything. It takes two to make a house a home.

When Mike comes home on payday, he is eager to lay out the budget for the week, making sure that we each have a little something in our pockets after each category is met. Budget meeting for us is a happy time since it gives us a feeling of accomplishment. The money is available in advance, not already spent before we even get it like it used to be. We make less than half the pay now but feel twice as rich since we restructured our lives.

Feeling secure is important, but one of the most important ways I need my husband is to remember that life is about play and enjoyment. Getting all of our work done is a lot more fun when we do it together. Similarly, doing housework while he is on a job is more fun because I know he will be surprised when he sees what I did in his absence. I am inspired to get more done just to hear him say, "Wow! How did you do all of that? You're a tough guy!" I feel light and energized by his gratitude and he feels the same way because I appreciate what he does.

It is not that I feel pressured to earn his respect but when he expresses his love for me, I know it is genuine. There is no question that he needs me and that his life is better with me. Multiply that by two and you get what I mean.

BUTCHER BLOCK COUNTERTOPS

Mike made me a temporary countertop for an old, heavy white porcelain sink he rescued from a demolition that requires more than just a plywood countertop. When I asked him to get my sink going so I could actually stand up to wash dishes, I didn't understand how solid the temporary set-up would have to be.

What happened is that our temporary countertops look so good, we have been tempted to keep them. What I like about using the 4X4 hardwood scraps that were used as skids for our building materials is that they aren't perfect. That means I don't have to be overly protective of the countertops in the kitchen. I have found that any imperfection caused due to my reckless use can be easily sanded down and refinished with some Tung oil.

So, here's how we did it. You line up the required number of 4X4's or whatever you have, making sure that they are equally thick and equally long. Clean and sand any ground-in dirt so the glue will adhere. Measure out where your sink goes and mark it so you can cut it with a saws-all to get the curves of the corners right.

When you have your lumber all lined up the way you want it, take a pencil and mark lines so that you make sure when you cut out the pockets for the biscuit joinery that the pieces all assemble properly. This will indicate where to place the pockets for your wooden biscuits. You will need a biscuit cutter for this. I am pretty sure you could also use a drill and doweling to do the same thing.

Cut little pockets in each side of each board, making sure to keep everything in alignment so you end up with a smooth top. We used long clamps to keep our boards flat. Use wood glue in the pockets and connecting edges. Don't overdo it to avoid more sanding than needed. Finish with Tung oil.

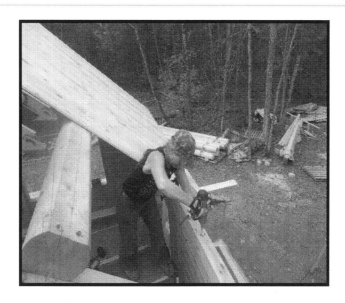

5. LIBRARY NIGHT
October 16, 2013

I like to touch books. For a number of reasons, my husband and I visit the tiny library in our local town at least once a week, usually twice. The first time we went there it was for the heat. We must have been a sight with our mismatched layers and uncombed hair after camping for a week in mid-February. I will never forget the welcoming smiles, the comfy chair, and of course, the familiar smell of books. The colorful jackets of new books wrapped in fresh, glossy covers renewed my spirits and made me feel at home. The two librarians appeared perfectly willing to pause in their business to welcome us and get to know what we like to read.

Kathy, observing that we were both new to the state, showed us the Maine shelf. My husband went straight for the non-fiction section and found two books. I just ran my hand up and down the rows, reading the titles slowly, marveling at how many books have been written. The sheer number overwhelms me sometimes and I get a sense of being in a crowded cocktail party where everyone is speaking but I can't make out any one thought. I am a slower reader. It takes me time to find a book, kind of like having a friend. It takes me time. I appreciate people and am friendly, don't get me wrong, but it takes me a long time to settle into a friend. Like my friends, my books become an integral part of my life.

"A lot of people really enjoyed this one," Kathy was noticing my inability to choose a book. She handed me a three-inch thick, white one with a quaint New England sketch of a farmstead in the winter on the cover. It was wrapped in clear plastic to preserve its beauty and there was a cheerful aspect to its appearance. It felt nice to touch something so clean and crisp. But I could tell it wasn't a new book since the pages were printed on thick paper.

"Hmm... *The Old Squire's Farm*," I said, "sounds enticing, I'll give it a try." That's another thing about me, I will try just about anything that comes highly recommended.

Kathy was right. C. A. Stephens' *The Old Squire's Farm* was a perfect delight to read. In fact, Mike and I both read it and then read parts out loud to each other and giggled at the antics of its characters. Reading aloud to each other has become a wonderful pastime for us since we have no television and no internet.

Library night has also become a favorite pastime for us for the same reasons. It gives us time to visit with our library friends and to try new things. It also gives us time to thaw out and rest in a comfy chair, research questions that have been brewing in our minds, and catch up on emails and social media. My job has been to post the pictures of our progress on the building of the house. This holds special importance after we have had a work party. It gives us a chance to share our appreciation with friends.

Some library nights we get caught up in our computer life and forget about the books. Working ten to fourteen hour days leaves me physically spent at the end of the day so I usually fall asleep after the first paragraph of a new book, very often ending my night with a pleasant thump as my hands give way and the book lands on my face.

We reluctantly returned *The Old Squire's Farm* and I avoided the Maine books for a while, thinking that nothing else could take the place of this wonderful new friend we had made. I checked out the Wednesday night book club choice, *The Unlikely Pilgrimage of Harold Fry* by Rachel Joyce and I read the entire book out loud to Mike. We followed Harold's journey as though it was our own, cheering him on when he needed it most. We would say to each other the next day, "remember when Harold…" to cheer ourselves on when *we* needed it most.

As the leaves turned and the acorns dropped, the days closed in on us and our timeline became more and more pressing to become weather-tight, we relished the thought of cuddling up in bed and hearing what happened next to our dear friend Harold. He had been through so much.

Returning *The Unlikely Pilgrimage of Harold Fry* was easy because we were eager for others to travel the road with Harold. You can't keep that kind of friendship to yourself. A pilgrim belongs to no one.

After Harold, I thought about returning to the Old Squire. It might be fun to visit with his rascally crew of orphaned grandchildren who solved their problems in quirky little ways. They were fun and we needed a little bit of that after the long road with Harold.

So, I returned to the Maine shelves on our next library night and my hands ran up and down the spines of each tome, reading through each title as though sight-seeing in a new country. Each book a little house or a large imposing homestead with lights on and people inside living stories of their own. One spine caught my hand, the way that a low branch might catch you and make you pause as you walk through the woods. "Here," it seemed to be saying, "is something you need to see."

It was an old brown book and I couldn't read the title from the spine. "Not a very popular one," I thought, "or Kathy would have covered it with clear plastic like the others." I pulled it out. In spite of loving to try good recommendations, I relish my own discoveries. And there it was.

Though words have always been my tools of trade, I pause in my ability to craft for you the exact emotion I felt when I held that old brown book in my hand. It was as though I had walked through the gates of time and was sitting in the old green chair of my grandparents' house. I could smell the coffee, cigarettes, and burnt toast mingled with the salty air and warm pines. This was a book I used to read in their house. My grandfather once remarked that it was unusual that I picked that book up again and again through my childhood. Maybe it was the pictures. I am not sure. It certainly wasn't the kind of book a child who roamed the beaches of Florida would be interested in. The author's tone was humorous and light but Louise Dickinson Rich wrote about living in the woods on the opposite end of the earth.

I loved Louise even back then. She had become a good friend with whom I lost touch over the years. My grandparents eventually sold their house and most of their books were donated. I spent many library days of my life searching for that book again, remembering what it looked like but nothing else, not even its title, *We Took to the Woods*.

There it was. What I had searched for my entire life, finally found me. I had to just wait until the time was right.

"Wow!" I couldn't contain myself, "I used to read this book at my grandparents' house." Kathy looked up. Funny thing about bookish types, they get the magic. Her eyes twinkled.

"I never even knew that was there. Hasn't been checked out in over ten years."

Mike and often remark about how wonderful it is to open a library book and see the little register in the back with dates stamped in it and a pocket for its card. It is an old system but our library still uses it. Of course, our tiny library also keeps books that haven't been checked out in over ten years.

As amazing and fantastic as my discovery was, I could not read Louise's book. Being about four inches thick, it hit hard at night when I dropped it on my face. Mike is the one who read it first.

"You'll like this book, Miche, Louise is a lot like you." He commented.

So one day when Mike went off to work and I was feeling a bit rudderless, I decided to stay in bed and just read *We Took to the Woods*. That night I read Louise's story out loud to Mike and we laughed and giggled at her wonderful voice. She had been a high school English teacher and decided to move to Northern Maine to live with her husband Ralph.

There wasn't an "Off-the Grid" subject line for her book. She wrote her story in the 1930's. Her neighbors were bears and transient loggers. But she saw life as a playground and approached everything with laughter, even giving birth to her only son by herself since there was no time to get the doctor.

Louise, I must tell you, is a remarkable woman. But, I have to be honest, I have kept her to myself for more than three months now.

"Going to have to check that book out again," I tell Kathy on another visit to the library. She understands. I consider searching for it on Amazon but it's *this* book I need to hold. It is part of my story now and Louise is my wise old friend, helping me find my way through the journey of my life and all of the words that go with it.

Strangely enough, a few months later, I received a thin package in the mail from the Head of the English department in Rhode Island. Enclosed was a heartfelt letter of recommendation, a touching card congratulating me on my move, and, in an uncanny twist of fate, a new paperback edition of *We Took to the Woods*.

I guess I can return my library book now.

LOUISE'S BAKED BEANS
(First hers, then mine, now yours.)

I have discovered why baked beans are such a staple up here in Northern Maine. You can make something nutrient rich with things that can remain on a dry shelf for a very long time and then set it on a wood stove for as long as you need to before they're eaten without ever having to refrigerate anything. You just keep adding water to them when they dry out. I add bacon to ours for flavor and calories. I have also added chourico, Portuguese pork sausage, because my husband likes it in just about everything, including cabbage and corned beef. One of these days, we will make our own chourico and it will appear in our next book.

If you haven't already set up a couple of 16 ounce jars of Northern white or Navy beans (see this how-to in Book II), take a pound of beans and pressure cook them. Louise is a stickler for baking her beans the whole way through from soaked raw to finished product. I don't have an oven in my wood stove, just a top, so I can't do that. You'll have to make your own adjustments based on what you've got as well.

Mix in about 1/3 cup molasses, ½ cup or so brown sugar, some dried mustard (1 tablespoon or so), pinch of salt, sautéed onion, and some cooked up chopped bacon. Pour it in a cast iron pot with lid and set it on the front of the wood stove and let it go for most of the day, checking for moisture and switch to the back of the stove.

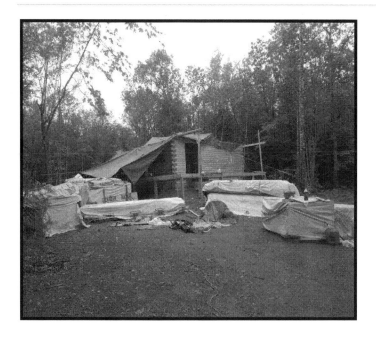

6. LIVING IN PARADISE
October 29, 2013

This, I consider, is not everyone's view of paradise. I don't quite understand why not, but I get it. A lot of people want to visit the country but they wouldn't want to live there. I feel the same way about New York City. There is a wonderful energy there that sweeps you up and says, "go see… there is so much to see!" I have always thought that one day I would enjoy a penthouse apartment in Manhattan. I picture myself like Holly Golightly, perusing the magically illuminated glass shelves of Tiffanies for breakfast. I am sleek and polished in a perfect black dress; my hair is in a perfect up-do and I glide through the streets of the city while everyone stares.

It's a rare country woman who even owns a little black dress. Even if the weather allowed for a smart sleeveless number at the church picnic, you'd have to make sure you layered over it for the mosquitoes and black flies. Besides, everything you own smells like wood smoke. There is no such thing as a dry cleaner in the country. Not unless you want to go a few towns over so you can clean a dress that you really can't wear anyway. So, what's the point?

People don't stare at you in the country. They look at you and if they're talking to you, they look you in the eye. They don't much care what you're wearing, if you smell like wood smoke, or if your hair is always pulled back in a simple braid. They care about *you*. When a country person asks you how you are doing, they really want to know. They aren't thinking, "How am I going to efficiently ask for my coffee so I don't get people in line all riled up." They're thinking, "How can I help you?"

And when they help, they really help. Take, for instance, the time my husband and I had car trouble in the middle of February and drove it into the shop of an acquaintance. We hadn't really known Brian for long but he and his girlfriend invited us in to get warm. We made a meal together. He called all over town to find a part we needed, and since we wouldn't be able to get it until the next day, we ended up staying at their place. He even offered to buy the part for us because we didn't have the cash. We sent him the check when we got home.

Or the time some other friends traveled down a logging road by accident in their truck camper and got stuck in the middle of mud season. We all showed up to help, using come-a-longs and straps and getting darn near flattened by the truck tire. We all shared in the disaster and to this day, it gives us something to laugh about. Since the heavy vehicle went off the side of the road and dug itself into a ditch, we weren't very successful that day. But as luck would have it, a logging truck (they don't travel down those roads in mud season – no one does), happened to pass by. After a couple of chuckles at our predicament, the logger said, "Wait here for forty-five minutes and I will be back." He did come back and hauled our friends' truck camper right out of the ditch, with hardly a scratch.

That's the way things are in the country. We gave him some home baked cookies and a jar of our honey and he was happy to have helped.

It's not uncommon for a tradesman to come out to do an estimate and ask, "Let's see, it will be this much," he pointed to the bill, "but I'll see what I can do. Does your wife bake cookies?" Little things carry a lot of weight out here. Cookies can save the job or sharpen the pencil on an estimate. Two dozen cookies have bought us half a yard of good composted loam for our garden or a hand with setting up the plumbing.

Things like saying "Good morning" and being able to talk to people about what's on your mind are important here. For the most part, people don't care where you stand but they want to know. And if you are unfair in your transactions, word gets around and fair people won't even come out for an estimate. There's a pure logic in the way people do business here.

I guess a person's idea of paradise all boils down to what matters most to them. For some, being able to go to a museum at will and try the latest in fashion and cuisine is important. For me, it's being recognized at my bank, joking around with the cashiers at the food market, and finding fellowship in a small church. It's about being able to say to someone, "Hey, I can help with that, I have a log-splitter that I am not using right now. I'll bring it over next Tuesday and we'll get your wood set up for winter."

Paradise to me is also about drinking clean water and breathing good fresh air that has been filtered through millions of trees. It is about fresh unprocessed milk and eggs and vegetables bought from people who grew them. To me it is about looking people in the eye when you talk to them and recognizing that everyone here is struggling in some small way and understanding that no life is perfect.

No life is ever completely together, no matter how groomed and clean a person's appearance. The same problems exist in the lithe little figure of Holly G. having *Breakfast at Tiffany's* as in Beth S. in her sweatshirt who sets the deep fryer every morning at the gas station, drinking her coffee out of a Styrofoam cup. When you boil down the whole human experience, it doesn't matter whether you are a country mouse or a city mouse, all you want is a little cheese and someone to love. It's pretty simple.

For some, paradise is being able to find their cheese in the woods and fields around them. For others, it means being able to find their cheese 24-7 right around the corner in a little coffee shop. Either way, getting the cheese requires some effort and risks.

For me, the risk of losing my deeper insights in all of the racket and clutter of a city scape doesn't seem worth the kind of processed and imported cheese you can get in the city. It costs too much.

As far as the breakfast of gloss and glitter in the Tiffany's showcase, I think it pales in comparison to the way the river glistens liquid silver with diamond accents when the sun's rays hit it at just the right angle around tea time. Whether in the city or the country, this kind of magic reveals itself to those who are willing to pause on occasion. Perhaps this ability is the only key we need to find paradise.

Bzzzz...OFF: AKA: PARADISE LOST

Around these parts, our town is known for its trestle bridge over the river, its dirt road and potholes, its small population and a single stop sign. To be honest, even around here, most people don't even know where our town is. Our town is, however, famous with U. Maine's entomologists because it's considered the best place in Maine to study the black fly.

That's bragging rights, I'll tell you. One of my favorite T-shirts of all time reads: "Black flies: defenders of the wilderness since 1806!" It's true. It takes a certain mettle to remain calm when they crowd your space. They actually bite too. It's not a sting like mosquitoes, it's a chunk of flesh missing and a streak of blood dripping from the little laceration. Sounds ghastly. Trust me, it is.

That's why you'll see most black fly neophytes flailing their arms about in a desperate dance of hysteria reminiscent of King Kong on the top of the Empire State Building. Truth is, eventually you realize that the more heated you get, the more they swarm around you. Stay calm and they lose interest, unless of course, you're the only bait in town.

Even the young contractors who were raised to laugh in the face of this dark foe, the boys who scoffed at my initial offerings of *Bzzzz-Off*, were requesting it within two days of digging our foundation in mid-August. The stuff works.

Most of my recipes are the result of an accidental happenstance of some sort. I created Bzzzz-Off when I thought having my family camp out with us while we did the ground-breaking would be a good idea. It would be a celebration of my 50th birthday and they could help out with the building.

Being the obvious rookie that I was, I had no idea what torture a ground-breaking entails, but picture this: It is mid-July and people's cars are all jammed into our muddy (did I mention mud season?), tree-lined driveway, large trucks are waiting for the mud to dry up to get in, and to top it all off, it's the HEIGHT of Black Fly season and we have no house to dart into.

I needed to come up with something really fast.

Spray Bottle Insect Repellent
4 oz. witch hazel
18 drops each: lavender, citronella, cedar, wintergreen
essential oils

Salve or Stick Insect Repellent
¼ cup coconut oil
¼ cup Shea butter
¼ cup beeswax
40 drops each: vitamin e oil, citronella, tea tree, lavender,
cedar, wintergreen essential oils

The spray bottle is helpful to keep the dark cloud of aggressors at bay so you can get a grip as you reach for the salve. For long-term peace and tranquility, use the salve.

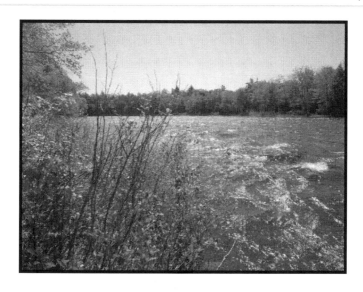

7. LISTENING TO SILENCE
October 31, 2013

While Mike is away at work, I have gained a new appreciation for spending all day with my own thoughts. I can see why some might go a little batty in solitude. Being alone for extended periods can force you to pay attention to the bats in the belfry. Most minds have closets and corners that are infrequently visited and must be dusted out.

For close to thirty years as a flooring contractor, Mike has had to spend the majority of his days working alone. He started out with a crew but as money got tighter, he had to let them go, one-by-one. Eventually, he was left with only his own thoughts to keep him company all day long. As a high school teacher, I shared the company and thoughts of hundreds of people. In many ways, his daily experience was the complete antithesis of mine. I often thought I would go batty with all of the noise and the distraction of my day. In some ways, I did.

I never considered how difficult his day of solitude might have been over the chaos of my own fractured mind. He would often claim that I was not really listening to him when he spoke and this was true. I had developed a method of scanning lightly through all of the noise and would not focus entirely on any one thought. It's a common process, akin to seeing the forest but not the trees. It made for some pretty funny conversations that would always end in, "I just told you that ten minutes ago." That comment from him made me feel a lot like my students. And, a little batty.

I think I passed the threshold into the realm of batty this week while I worked alone on the house. I walked through the front door of my brain, wandered around it, going from one room in my mind to another and finally decided that I don't think I want to stay in these dusty old places of my mind. I didn't exit running, but almost.

Don't get me wrong. I am not saying I need to return to the hundred-voiced chaos of my teaching days to find some peace of mind. What I am saying is that my alone time, time with my own thoughts, has afforded me the opportunity to sort through the lingering notions of my ordinary brain and say, "Yes, I know you have been there all along," and "No, I haven't really been listening, I was scanning again. Sorry."

"It's okay." The little thought says and then stews in the corner until it gets an attitude and won't come out again. After a number of years, the corners of your mind get stuffed with all of these little thoughts that you never paid any attention to and they are all shrieking to get out of the corner the minute you turn off the scanner and you allow silence. It's a crazed dance into the realm of Shame and Blame, over-lorded by Doubt, that demonic force that undermines the confidence of any happy person.

In short, it will drive you batty if you let it.

Fortunately, I was able to sort through all of the shadows of doubt, get in there and dust out the sticky cobwebs that build up over the years. Brains get especially dusty when you add in other people's opinions. The sticky web of its drama can grab you and pull you in. It's a dark world that I prefer to avoid by keeping a cheerful disposition. But when left alone with my thoughts, I can't avoid it. I have to get back into those closets and sort through, throw out, and clean up. It's a project.

Out here with no distractions, no traffic sounds, nothing

but the peaceful song of the river and my sunbathing dog to keep me company, I have the space and time to sort through those shadowy corners. I am free to feel each emotion completely, face the doubts and quietly discuss them in a reasonable tone without shame and blame getting in on the mix. I can sort through my memories (not all of them *pleasant misty-colored memories*) and put them in order.

Being alone with my own thoughts has been a little painful sometimes. But I think I have made it out the other end more sane and content with myself than I was when I entered. It's kind of like that House of Horrors that you hate while you are experiencing it, but feel somehow better afterwards. They are, after all, simply fake cobwebs in the corners. Just like the ghosts in the haunted house are only college kids wearing white make-up and sheets. Most of what our brains conjure up are purely experiences we'd rather not revisit that have been sulking in the corners of our minds so long they become inflated and ghostly with the lack of sun.

Like any little demon, if you face it, let it have its say and allow it to move on, it won't hurt you. In nature, bats serve a really good purpose, dispatching mosquitoes by the handfuls, but they don't belong in your belfry. Silence, time, space, and truth are like mighty shop-vacs, clearing out those dusty corners, giving those bats a reason to move on.

MARY JANES
(Our Favorite Construction Cookie)

Just for the record, there is nothing illicit or hidden in these cookies but they will make you hungry. We named them after one of my creative cooking experiments went wild. I was trying to make a healthier peanut butter cookie. We discovered that these cookies taste just like the little brown Mary Jane candy that trick-or-treaters still get in their pillow case bags every Halloween. You might recognize them; their packaging hasn't changed since we were kids in the Sixties. They are still wrapped in a golden-yellow wax paper with a red stripe down one side. Mike and I discovered that we are probably the only two people in this country that prefer Mary Janes to any other candy and we could only get them by pilfering our kids' Halloween stashes. This hasn't happened in a while so it felt nostalgic when we tasted this accidental cookie. We both recognized the flavor immediately.

Mix together a couple of pats of butter and just under a half-cup of coconut oil. It's easier to work with if you melt it first. Half-cup peanut butter, ½ cup brown sugar, a little under a ¼ cup molasses, 1 egg, 2 cups flour, scant ¼ cup coconut flour, ½ teaspoon baking soda, ½ teaspoon baking powder. Make little balls, flatten with a fork in two directions just like you do peanut butter cookies. Bake at 375 degrees for nine minutes. Cool before eating if you can wait. Great with cold milk.

We might be too old for trick-or-treating but we're never too old for milk and cookies!

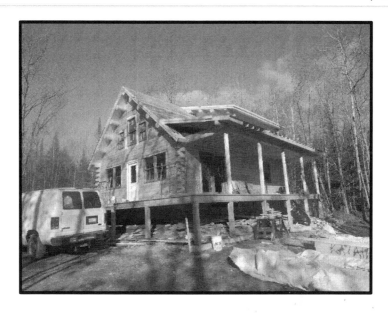

8. WALKING IN GRATITUDE
November 26, 2013

Living a life of simplicity (some might call it "living without") requires a person to be resourceful. I have found the old adage to be true: the mother of my most ingenious moments were when I found myself in the most necessity. This is how I discovered what a wonderful tea sweet fern makes. I knew it was used medicinally in salves to calm itchy, irritated skin, but I had no clue how it truly lives up to its name and makes my tea naturally sweet. I find it mixes well with other plants from the woods such as the simple but beautiful goldenrod, yarrow flower, and white pine needles. I added a smidge of cinnamon and made up a tasty late fall and winter tea without spending more than the dime the ground cinnamon cost.

It warms me twice because of the appreciative smile I get from my husband when I share it with him. Truly the short story of my sweet fern discovery began with two roads in the woods when confronted with an inability to purchase the herbs

I normally use for my nighttime teas. I could have chosen the road of doing without, but I chose the road of gratitude and that made the difference between simply surviving and truly thriving. I took a foraging hike instead of a car ride to town and examined my resources. By listening to the plants, watching for how they greeted me as I appreciated their beauty, I gathered a goodly supply of herbal tea for the winter. It took a little previous knowledge (mostly from friends) and some back-up research to check and double check for safety, but I ended up with a perfect tea blend and the memory of a delightful autumn afternoon of hiking in each cup.

The same sort of unusual adventuring has led to some of my more amusing inventions like the "tuna candles" I made one year because I needed candles for camping. I had a lot of tuna cans for some reason and an annoying collection of half-burned candles that ran out of wick before the paraffin. I cut strands from a cotton mop for new wicks, melted the wax, and created longer-lasting votive candles that made my friends laugh. It was definitely worth the time.

While I am on the subject of light, I have to mention the oil lamps Mike and I learned how to make in Pennsylvania (see how-to in another chapter) There are a growing number of people who make it their hobby and sometimes, their missions, to keep knowledge of how to do things alive. They are more than happy to learn and share how things were done before we could just pop down to the dollar store and pick up a battery-operated lantern.

Take socks as an example. It took me over a year of asking but I finally figured out how to knit my first pair. Most people think it's ridiculous to spend time and money on knitting socks when you can get them so cheaply in town. True. But there is nothing quite as satisfying as a handmade pair of wool socks.

Sometimes it's the gratitude that leads us into inventing the best things. While out foraging for blackberries last fall, we couldn't help but notice all of the wonderful milkweed pods in the same area. Knowing that if you pick them when they are less than two inches, they make a wonderful vegetable, Mike and I wondered if we could also harvest them and can them.

Milkweed pods taste just like green beans when they are cooked so we decided to try and preserve them in a hot pickle brine. Since the purple onions were ready in my garden, I threw a few chunks of those in for color and interest (as though a milkweed pod pickle isn't interesting enough).

Mother Nature was incredibly bountiful this fall and being grateful for her gifts has led us into some great discoveries. Being outside and harvesting her offerings led me to the conclusion that the winter might be a little long and cold up here. Thinking about our conversations about gratitude and foraging with our friends, Heather and Glenn, I noticed that being grateful for nature's gifts inevitably leads me to even more of her gifts. I noticed that the minute I took the time to bend down to pick blueberries, the more I saw to harvest. The gifts came in greater number when I was grateful and didn't just pass them by.

Some gifts are good just for grazing, others for collecting. Nothing beats the ability to chew on a winterberry leaf (wintergreen) while out in the woods. One day, when I have figured out how best to use them, I will harvest them too. But for now, I still delight in finding the little waxy pink berry and chewing on a leaf as I walk.

Now, when I go for a walk in the woods, I carry my foraging basket. I don't know what I am looking for but if I go out with a grateful eye, I am bound to find something good.

HOT PICKLED MILKWEED PODS

There's a latex sap that gives this wonderful plant its name. You have seen it growing wild in fields all across the country. Its pods turn brown at the end of the warmer months and release a silky, white seed that blows around in the wind. There are purple milkweed plants that aren't to be used and **never** use the pod when it gets old enough to show a brown or black seed. Stay safe and harvest the seed pods when they are under two inches in length and they are a nice light green color, white and silky inside with tender white seeds, if any. An easy system to check is only harvest light green pods smaller than your thumb.

Before using the pods for anything, always boil the pods for at least ten minutes and discard the water to remove its milky sap. They won't kill you if you eat them raw but some people get a little stomach ache from them. I never have felt queasy from eating them raw but I'm also not tempted to eat too many of them in the field. One pod always seems to be enough. Boiled pods taste just like green beans. I tried pickling them like you would okra pods and they came out really tasty. I especially appreciated them in mid-winter when good, fresh greens are hard to get. I mixed them with my sprouts for an easy salad; it already comes dressed in a vinaigrette dressing.

Take your pods, chopped onion (red looks pretty), whole garlic, and your typical canning liquid for pickling with ¼ cup of crushed red pepper. Pickling liquid is usually 4 cups water, 8 cups vinegar (I prefer cider), 1 cup sugar, 2 tablespoons salt. Water bath can for 15 minutes.

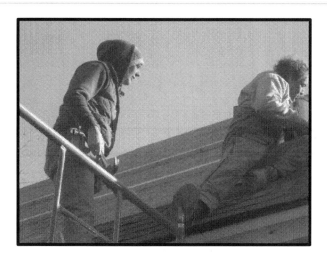

9. SURVIVING?
December 8, 2013

As any student of culture will tell you, the key difference between thriving and surviving has always been the evidence of creativity. I wonder if it is more like the chicken and the egg theory. Is it, as most cultural theorists will assert, that the only way people can be creative is to have their basic needs met with a generous margin of error? Or, I wonder, is it more likely that when forced to meet their basic needs, people must be creative?

I lean in the direction of the latter since it takes creativity to survive.

"So girl, how are you doing?" my father asked me a few weeks back.

"Fine. Just working hard to get weather-tight by the first snow fall." The crack in my voice was evident since Mother Nature's deadlines are real deal-breakers. There's no negotiating with her. We were cutting it close, still living in a camper with no heat and a frozen water system.

"I get it, just surviving," he said.

"Yes, I guess so." It had been a long day and I was tired

and in no mood for explanations.

After saying my goodbyes, I thought, I probably should have told him that even though I was physically fatigued, hungry for a good meal, and in desperate need of a long, hot shower, I was in no way simply surviving.

Surviving, I thought, was when I had to force myself to go to a job that was affording me less and less of my own autonomy and was choking out my daily expressions of creativity. Surviving was what I went through every hour of that day, yearning to be able to be right where I am now. Though my basic needs are not met with a large margin of error, I am free to be as creative as I choose. In fact, it is essential for my survival that I am creative. That, I strongly believe, is the difference between surviving and thriving.

As I meet other people who live off the grid, who homestead, or just simplify, there is a commonality that they all share. First, and foremost, they treasure their freedom. They are free to create the life of their choosing, whether it be to live in a $6,000 house with more cracks in it than an elephant's hide or they possess a ten-acre homestead with every type of cultivated flora and fauna useful to both man and woman. Whatever problems they encounter in their chosen walks of life, they are free to solve their problems their own way, applying their own God-given right to be creative.

"I believe that we are created in His image. That means we are supposed to be like Him," commented a young Baptist minister on the subject of creativity. We were working together on a customer's kitchen and were talking about literature. I couldn't agree with him more. Creativity is our trail marker when climbing closer to expressing the God-head in us all.

In the world of mundane existence, our creativity is constantly being thwarted by others who have control over us. If it doesn't fit the team goal or no one else "gets it," our own freedom to be creative can be sentenced to solitary confinement. If we are lucky, we might figure out a way to channel it into something like a knitting circle that is acceptable (or considered a waste of time by some).

So very often I have heard a friend say, "I am not the creative type."

That just bugs me. Yes, you are. Everyone is creative. It is just that when we are forced to solve our problems the same way everyone else does, or better yet, are not allowed to even have any problems, well, you see what I mean. There is a certain lack of freedom in that whole equation. It's the same equation that incarcerated your creativity. It might be comfortable to live in that place. You might have a hot shower at the end of a long day, but guaranteed, you are going to need one because there is some part of your essence that is being shut off and you might only get a day pass with no conjugal privileges if you get too wrapped up in the world of comfort and conformity.

Simply put, you're just not thriving. I know. I have lived in that place for most of my life. I have dreamed of one day being free to just create my day as I choose.

So, when I meet other so-called survivalists, I look into their faces and see the light of an individual. I see a gruff exterior, sometimes a little unwashed, perhaps wearing patched-up clothing and no particular hairstyle, but I also see beautiful hand-made hats, leggings, feather earrings, new ways to use objects such as a scarf for a skirt. I see combinations of colors and textures and babies that are wrapped up in their mother's arms rather than in a mechanical contraption with six moving parts.

Thriving is harvesting the bounty of nature. It is knowing how delicious milkweed pods are and then creating a new recipe to pickle them. It is being able to stop in the middle of some task and look up to spot a bald eagle flying overhead. It is the joy of cracking open your own blackberry jam that you foraged and canned with a friend. It is the surprise you get when the walnuts you picked and processed were all stolen by the squirrels one night because you left them out by accident.

Thriving is knowing that if you feel the need to stay in bed an hour longer, you won't get a "talking to" by your boss the next day. It is waking up early and getting started on something when the time is right, when the weather permits, when it should get done. It is not the panic you feel when you really want to stay at home on a cold icy morning and are running late and your windshield is all iced up. And creative expression cannot be limited to what color shirt and tie combination you would like to wear today.

Thriving is about giving creativity its place in your life. It is about recognizing that life is full of problems that must be solved on a daily basis but when given the freedom to be creative, these problems become our friends, not our enemies. It's okay to have problems; it's actually normal.

Too often, in the mundane world, the world of uber-conformity, problems are not our friends. They are things we are supposed to leave at home. There is no room in the workplace cubicle for them. Any problems must be submitted to the committee for review. Any solution will have to be done by committee agreement. Any individual ideas must be agreed upon and then they become the committee's ideas.

People I meet out here who would rather live in an old house with a million issues and no electricity get to take credit for their own ideas. If they are lamed-brained, so be it. They are free to live out the results of their own solutions, even if it means a mighty cold winter with lots of layers of wool (and hand-made socks do keep you warmer). It's not so bad, they'll tell you. And truly, what do I care, other than to offer a little assistance next fall to help them better weather-tight their home.

"We can wrap your house with all of these tarps we have extra that covered the wood we used for building our house," I tell my friends. We agree that it is a good use for something other people might just throw away.

It makes for a great day of friendship, working together to chink up all of the cracks with loose insulation, spray foam, and then tacking down the recycled black tarps. When we got a text message with a picture of his digital thermometer later that week that read 15 degrees exterior, 88 interior temperature, we laughed. All it took was a little time and some creative problem-solving to make four people really happy this winter. It didn't take a committee. And, either way, we are all free to thrive while surviving, even if sometimes it is with a low margin of error.

TWO USEFUL PLANTS FOR WINTER TEA

Sweet fern is a low bush that looks a lot like a fern but isn't. It appears in late spring, summer, and fall in New England. It likes to grow in inhospitably dry and gravelly soil so, like most great plants, loves road-sides. Rule of thumb is to avoid road-sides as dangerous places for a number of reasons. All foragers say that plants in those soils absorb the grunge and fumes of passing cars. So, use your judgment and try to find them in less-travelled places.

The roadside can be helpful for plant ID. Then, the plants will educate you and you'll learn to see them where you never noticed them before. It's a lovely process that becomes a communication between human and plant that you can only experience by being quiet and willing to really appreciate the beauty around you. That's a little hard to do on some heavily-travelled road-sides so take some secondary routes for a change.

So, why sweet fern? The leaves are typically used in an oil infusion and mixed with a base to make a great skin salve. It calms and soothes dry rashes like sunburn but is also good for oily itches like poison ivy, and toxic-type itches like bug bites. It also, true to its name, is a great sweetener for your teas and retains its properties when ingested, being a good stomach tonic like mint or juniper.

It grows in large swaths so there is no danger of over-harvesting, unless of course, you live up to the name the Native Americans gave some European settlers, "wasichu." This term translates as "insatiably greedy people." I think we are beginning to see where that behavior leads.

White pine has similar benefits. The amazing thing about a tea made from the little brushy clumps of white pine tea is that it provides a generous amount of vitamin C.

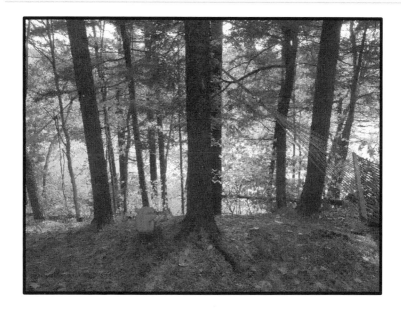

10. FINDING PEACE
December 9, 2013

Thinking about what we have found out here on the edge of the civilized world, I would have to say it is a certain peace. Some might argue that we are merely out of touch, that since we check our mail, both electronic and post office box, only once a week or so. I would have to reply we are in touch, just with something a little different, something pretty important.

There is a certain anxiety and lack of peace amongst men and women worldwide. More than ever, the world is on fire. Wars and disputes are being waged and fought at warp speed. Terrorizing citizens has become a hobby for some gangs here at home. Our country's leadership sends its young men and women all over the world on "peace missions" that are often far from peaceful. Technology has added a new level to the anxiety that all of this causes. With the advent of drones, the proliferation of countries that now have nuclear programs, and a growing concern for religious freedom, the reasons to feel anxious mount.

With all of this world-breaking news circulating constantly, it seems to me that the best thing that Mike and I can do about it is to settle into a little spot of peace. Perhaps, more than ever, our job is to demonstrate the possibility of peace. Or, more importantly, we might serve as the concrete example of the ability to wish for peace and then find it. In many ways, we are both refugees from the land of war. We have fought the battle for what we believed was good in our lives, families, communities, and even our country. We both have experienced self-abuse, relationship abuse, financial, and work-place abuse. We both have fought back, been involved, sought therapy, quit habits, taught, coached, volunteered, and campaigned for goodness and reason.

Looking back now, it seems to me that some of our efforts were successful but joining in the fight might be less effective in the long run than retreating into peace. Perhaps our most important fight yet is to simply stop playing the game of conflict. Perhaps our job now is to live in peace.

Living in peace with our surroundings and listening to the song of the river seems to be the most important job I have right now. I am not sure where it will lead but I know it is the right path. My entire being tells me so.

I have to admit that when I awaken at 6:30 and don't feel compelled to rush out the door with a coffee in my hand, I feel a little bit of survivor guilt. Sunday nights are delightful to me now since I know I will be working on what I want to accomplish on Monday morning, not what I am compelled to do. Mike and I call it "Fun-day" now.

If there is any urgency, it is a real urgency, caused by nature, my new boss. We have to button up the window bucks, stack the wood that is drying out in the front, can up the rest of the turkey soup, and Mike has to shore up the front wall of the house. We have work that must get done. We still don't have a shower. Our warm water comes from a big pot I put on the wood stove and we wash ourselves with that. We have almost everything we need to get that done so that's on the list for today. We definitely are busy. But we are not anxious.

I once watched an interview with the Dali Lama of Tibet about the concept of peace. One of the things he said is that Americans are always phrasing things in terms of a fight or a war. There's "a war on poverty", "a fight for the cure" and so many more that once you become aware of it, you begin to notice its ubiquitous nature.

Being peaceful is a choice we make. It takes constant awareness. Our brains are so programmed for conflict that we look for it if we are not careful. We look for it in the silliest places like a kitchen countertop that we just cleaned. Your husband comes along and places a cabbage on it right after you cleaned it and the conflict begins. There is no real reason to break up a peaceful day for it but it happens when you let your guard down.

If we step back and pay attention, we'll notice that through the mechanisms of popular culture, our brains are consistently being programmed for fear, doubt, and worry. These human emotions are fodder for news stations and advertisers (and a few other institutions I can think of too). In order to believe that peace can exist, we have to reprogram our minds. It takes constant effort and sometimes a little media fasting.

For some, living in a place where it would take the police and emergency vehicles about 40 minutes or so to reach their house is a scary idea. People ask us if we aren't worried about the bears, coyote, mountain lions, and strange folk in our neighborhood. I don't worry, I just take precautions. I carry my gun when I forage alone. I don't leave food out that might attract critters. I don't own anything of any value that someone else might want. I keep a few good fire extinguishers on hand. But most of all, I don't allow my mind to engage in fearful thoughts.

Whether it is in a bucolic small town or in a large messy city, there are always reasons to not feel peaceful. It is a state of mind. I just find it a little easier to find it out here where our newspaper and internet access is limited since we have no television and we get our news mostly when we go into town once a week. It doesn't completely stop the disruptions to my peace, but it slows it all down enough so I can still find it.

ST. JOHN'S WORT

If you recognize the name of this plant (*wort* is an Old English word for herb or flower), you probably already know what it is good for. It's a natural anti-depressant and mood elevator. Like most of Mother Nature's healers, it also possesses other beneficial qualities such as anti-inflammatory properties. Here's how to find it but be aware that when you harvest, leave the roots, unless you absolutely need them, and never take more than 1/3 of any given plant. Take from the outer growth, moving outer edge in to help the inner growth get sunlight, and leaving the older, middle branches, as plants have parent branches that are necessary for regrowth.

As always, avoid taking anything from road-sides (as mentioned previously). But, as our incredibly forgiving mother would have it, this is another plant that loves gravelly, dusty road- sides. Use the road-side to identify (quickly and carefully, I will add), and then you will begin to see this lovely, tall, and unassuming yellow flower everywhere. Its appearance belies its beautiful nature: ready to sprout anywhere things get rough, adding a cheerful grace to an otherwise dismal scene. This is true of so many beneficial plants but St. John's Wort has a bit of a disheveled attitude that, once you know it, you will recognize it anywhere in a row of wild flowers.

St. John's Wort has the unique bed-hair quality of a natural born charmer that says, "I don't have to try too hard to be wonderful. I just am." To identify: peer through its leaves towards the sun and you'll see what looks like tiny perforations in them; its stamen is a little brush of golden hairs.

So what do you do with St. John's Wort? Harvest its stems, leaves, and flowers in mid to late summer and use them to make a topical infusion in olive oil for any aches and pains, especially the joint-swelling kind. Believe me, it works. To make an oil infusion you have to soak the plant in oil for ten days at the magical body temperature of between 90 degrees and 110 degrees. Stir it all up a few times a day. The more you fuss with it, the better it will get. This is when using an electric yoghurt-maker comes in handy. Store all infusions in a light-resistant bottle (dark green, blue, or amber). To make mine, I use my Conservo and leave it on the deck in the sun.

To make a tincture, I like to use 1/3 Mason jar of grain alcohol (you can use a good vodka too) and 2/3 water to cover the plants and let sit in the dark for at least three months, shaking it on occasion. I haven't tried it yet but my friend Heather says she uses glycerin to make her tinctures. It's worth trying.

I make a St. John's Wort cordial by adding about ½ cup sugar to a 16 ounce mason jar, dissolving it in the water first, and then adding a few warming spices like allspice, nutmeg, and cardamom in whole seed form. Let the herbs steep for at least three months before you strain the cordial through a coffee filter. I have to say, it was nice to be able to share this warming mixture with guests when they stopped by this winter. I make cordials from other fruits and herbs but this one is my favorite because it is a true medicinal. Always take in small doses, of course.

I also allow the leaves and flowers of St. John's Wort to dry out for a soft addition to my winter tea. It is naturally good for seasonal depression disorder which can occur during a long and really cold winter. I'm happy I added some to my tea last fall. I am still smiling, even though it snowed again yesterday (April 14th). Thanks St. Johnny!

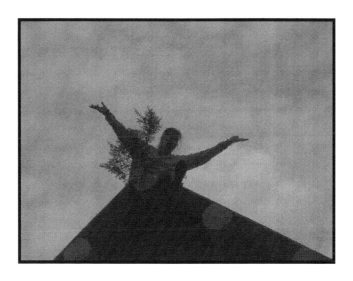

11. THE GOD SQUAD
December 11, 2013

When I was teaching high school English in Miami Beach years ago, I served as the advisor for the school's literary magazine. The year before I took over, there was a bit of controversy about the type of poetry the magazine was allowing students to publish. The hullabaloo was all about church and state and the separation of the two in a high school. The subject of the controversial poetry was God. The literary club had been inundated by Jesus Freaks that year and they couldn't help but write about their love for the Divine. There was an eclectic mix of Godly types on the staff those years, including a couple of Buddhist and Reformed Jews. I reasoned that the school's literary magazine had always published the dark and hellish poetry that is considered normal for American teenagers. Censoring the God-Squad poetry seemed like a clear double standard to me. Why shouldn't they be allowed to write and publish their love for Jesus and the Divine? My argument eventually settled the case. As it turns out, the God-Squad went on to win many Silver and Gold awards in the Columbia University annual competitions while they ran the magazine.

What I learned from that group of students was that faith can make a person strong. Since adolescents are heavily influenced by their peers, faith can be contagious. My magazine and newspaper staffs during those years were all bright-eyed, self-contained youths with a penchant for learning and a true respect for me, their peers, and themselves. At the time, I couldn't help but notice that even though they all dealt with the usual teenage stuff like broken homes (one was even in a foster-home), alcoholic parents, malnutrition, and weight and skin distractions, they seemed pretty darned healthy compared with most other teens. Back then my reasoning was simple. They worked hard. That was all I needed to know to have faith in them.

Their faith, I learned, made them resilient and productive. I have often thought about that group of kids when I have been confronted with the question of whether there is any credence to having faith in God. My experience is that if it makes you better able to deal with all of the complexities of life, it has to be good. God is good.

What my students taught me those years is that getting to know God isn't such a whacky thing. In fact, it's kind of cool. And, it works. Calling on Him when I am in an emotional fix has been a true life-saver in many ways. Thinking about emulating what Jesus stood for such as compassion, love, forgiveness, and mercy have been good for my character. Listening to songs about all of that stuff on the radio puts me in a really positive frame of mind and keeps me looking forward to my future with confidence. Faith, it seems, is the encouragement to believe that in spite of all of my obstacles along the way, everything is and will be okay. Learning to love Jesus doesn't mean that I didn't also want to love Buddha, though. There's room in my heart for both. Since I feel strongly about that, I'm pretty sure God's okay with it too.

Walking away from the life we had built full of mortgages and ready-made every-things to build our own house in the woods has been a journey of faith on many levels. It has been a pilgrimage of sorts. There is a Zen Buddhist saying that if you take the leap, the net will appear. I am grateful to my little God-Squad, Mike, my family, and my other teachers over the years who have helped me find my faith in the net because I have taken the leap. Doing so has made my life full of fun and useful surprises. As soon as you start to notice it, the synchronicity is astonishing. The more grateful I have been for the little gifts and messages I receive from the Universe, the more I praise the Great Creator for them, and the more they appear. It is a sweet way to live.

Take, for example, the fact that building a house requires a lot of specialized tools. As a flooring installer and over-all fixit-guy, Mike has many tools. But there were a lot of things we needed and couldn't afford to buy. Fortunately, our close friend worked in construction for many years before she became a science teacher. She brought a lot of important tools with her when she visited to help us build. Still, there was critical equipment we did not own. We told ourselves that we would figure it out. Purchasing them was out of the question and renting would be tough on the budget. It would set other projects back. We were strong in the faith that things would work out.

The first confirmation of our faith came when Mike's mom asked us to help her clean out her late husband's tool shed. We both truly loved Pops and he loved us too. We took on the job of cleaning out the shed with a certain amount of reverence since he had been a skilled and meticulous craftsman, as a boat captain for the owner of a large clothing manufacturer. When we opened the door to the tiny shed, we couldn't believe how he managed to fit so many tools into the shed in such an organized and useful manner. Every tool was well-maintained, in its original box, and within reach when he needed it.

What surprised us more than Pop's care and love of his tools was the fact that almost every tool in the shed was something we would be needing for the building of our house.

"Wonder why he has one of these?" Mike held up a router, and a set of forstner Bits.

"Can't tell you. I don't even know what those things are for," his mom replied.

We couldn't help but think that Pops was our little construction angel in Heaven making sure we could get our job done. Still there was so much more we would need. Our house wasn't selling in Rhode Island and we would have to figure out how we would be able to pay for the materials. For two years we had fashioned a chart shaped like a thermometer on the back of an old envelope and stuck it to our fridge. As we saved money, we filled in the thermometer. We planned our finances on making no money on the sale of the house. Looking back, it's a good thing we did because that's exactly what finally happened.

We would have to make-do, we reasoned. But we weren't going to let anything get in the way of our dream. We would work hard and make it happen.

Basically, we relied on faith that we would be able to build this thing together. We have what it takes, we told ourselves. We prayed together every night and at special moments that God would guide us in the right direction and that we would be of service to our families and whomever He wanted us to touch. Walking in the faith that we were following His guidance, we finally did come up with the money. We gathered the money bit by bit after two years and some decision-making about retirement funds. Our budget would be really tight. We would improvise the rest, we told each other.

But when it came to construction scaffolding, improvising is a dangerous enterprise. I had to look away more than a few times when Mike created his makeshift scaffolding, using ladders that are not meant to be separated and shim upon shim, while building the house. Praying to God for help at that moment was helpful in more than a few ways. My experience has been that He always listens and helps.

Mike likes to say, "God hates a coward." That statement is usually followed up with, "He doesn't much fancy fools either." Teetering on the edge of some precariously placed board that sags in the middle and looks like he borrowed the set-up from Dr. Seuss doesn't inspire even a smile from me.

But he managed to fall only once and survive it without

major damages. Building walls with this make-shift scaffolding was one thing, but when it came time for the roof, we were going to have to make some hard decisions about safety.

We didn't plan for accidents in our budgeting. We prayed for help.

Within a day of having the discussion about budgets and ways to make what we would need, Larry showed up.

Larry had been working on his new camp down the road from our property and was wrapping things up for the season. Being a contractor, Larry has replicates of all the tools required to build a house. He also has a uniquely generous and jovial nature. The combination of those two was exactly what we needed. But we had no clue how helpful Larry was going to be.

"Hey, I have all of this scaffolding and roofing equipment at camp, why don't you come over tomorrow and pick it all up. I'll help you unload. You can keep it through the winter since I won't be back up until then."

I am certain I could hear Pops up there chuckling. He and God must have been dancing a jig. It was all too uncanny.

What we found is that our faith has led us to some amazing experiences. The synchronistic events while building our house have been too numerous to write about here but one in particular touched us deeply.

Tragically, some years ago, Mike's younger brother, Ray, died in a fishing accident. The year before he died, he helped us move into our house in Rhode Island and he showed up with a roll of Blue Pex Tubing that is used for plumbing in very cold climates. It is expensive stuff but we really didn't need it since our house in Rhode Island was already built.

"Ray, I don't need this. It's just going to sit here and be the shed-spread Michele hates so much."

"Just keep it Moe. You're going to need it someday." And it sat in the back yard for about eight years, collecting other odds and ends of things that don't fit in the shed and don't serve any particular purpose other than to grow mosquito colonies.

The day a friend came over as a trade of carpet

installation for plumbing, we used the Blue Pex Tubing to set up our water lines. That's when Mike told me about Ray's comment. We both said a prayer for Ray and thanked him. We knew he was present at that moment in some way that we both admit we don't fully understand. Later that night Ray's picture fell out of the book Mike was reading before bed. Neither of us remembers putting it there.

While building our house, we have witnessed many answered prayers and synchronistic experiences that include appearances by friends and offers of help by people at just the right time. Each time it has strengthened our faith.

Mike recently read a book about Neuroplasticity that we both found interesting. The basic premise of that science is that we can determine which pathways in our brains become super-highways just through training ourselves to think certain thoughts. Naturally, if we build the fear and worry pathways, those neurons beg to be activated even if we don't have anything to worry about at the moment. Those negative pathways will demand attention, telling us that we need to worry. The way to channel this brain activity is to consciously create replacement pathways that lead to more positive outcomes. To me, that means pray more, think about God more, be grateful, love life and the people in my life, and have faith that even the difficult moments are ultimately good for me if I learn from them.

As we approach Christmas, we have found that because of building the house, we will not be with family and friends during the holidays but are content in the faith that we will be hosting a warm country Christmas for our family in the years to come. With no money to spend on Christmas presents, I had to engage in some creativity to make all of the presents for family members. I am happy in this predicament because I have in my heart the true meaning of Christmas. My little hand-made socks and trinkets are filled with love.

This Christmas, Mike and I will be going to church, volunteering for the community Christmas luncheon, and renewing our commitment to God to follow His plan. We also have been invited to some wonderful Christmas parties. One such party was at the house of a family that home-schools.

When we arrived at the family's house last Saturday night, we witnessed that all of the children were sledding down a homemade sled-slope that was all lit up like a ski slope. We were greeted by a family made of snow complete with a dog and skirt made out of pine boughs for the mother. We remarked at how creative the snow family was and how lovely it was for their parents to construct the sled-slope for their kids. We were wrong.

"Oh, no, the kids did that one day while I was out shopping. They borrowed their dad's tools and built the whole thing with lights and all while I was gone," their mother replied when we remarked at the wonder of the slope.

Later that night, the family and friends gathered for a little Bible study and prayer session. Imagine that? At a Christmas party? A smart young lady played Christmas carols on a piano and a group of children danced with each other in the living room. There were no children sneaking away to play Minecraft that night. They were present and active in the conversations. They were busy greeting guests, taking their coats, offering up snacks, and running in and out of the house with each other. I have to say, Mike and I were some of the happiest persons alive that weekend.

Mike and I always kid around that we like to shop a good sermon. This is true. When we are in conflict with each other or are feeling down about life, we look for a message to help us get through it. This was the case when we approached our two friends from the church of the Latter Day Saints. It was a cold February morning and I had been heavily stressing about our daughters. We were driving our car down the main street of our neighboring town when we spotted them. They were wearing identical down winter coats with fur-lined hoods, one tall and blonde, the other, brunette and of average height. They were obviously two young women on a mission.

"Maybe they have our message," Mike said.

"Okay, I'll approach them first; I don't want to startle them, after all, I'm sure they're not used to too many people seeking them," I said.

That was all it took to become good friend with Sister Dickson and Sister Burton, the same ages as our daughters and serving as missionaries from Utah. They indeed did have the message we needed: *Helaman 5:12* from *The Book of Mormon*: "...remember that it is upon the 'rock of our redeemer', who is Christ, the son of God, that ye must build your foundation... that when the devil hath sent forth his winds...it shall have no power over you..." The "devil" in our case, was doubt and fear that our girls would not have the strength they will need to survive this tough thing called life.

These two young ladies have a candid way of approaching ideas and discussing beliefs about God. I can honestly say that they have dispelled every preconceived notion I have held about Mormons and I find them pretty open and intelligent in their conversations. I also feel less anxious about my own two girls as I watch our two young friends brave the darkness and realize that we all must find our own paths in life. My faith in my girls is ultimately the best thing I can give them.

And so it seems that there's a new God Squad in town, providing me with fresh new ideas, ways to look at things, and a little hard work. Only this time, it is to help us build a log cabin in the woods as part of their service projects while they discuss their faith. Can't see anything wrong with that!

PIE-IN-THE-SKY PIZZA

I have always preferred to make my own pizzas. For one thing, it takes less time than locating the pizza delivery phone number, figuring out what everyone wants on it, ordering it from someone who can barely hear you, and then waiting so long for it to arrive that when it finally gets there, you're so starved you could care less what it tastes like or even is worth the twenty-something bucks you laid out for it.

And anyway, we can't get an emergency vehicle to come down here, far less a kid delivering pizza. Though we did a get a couple of Jehovah's Witnesses the day after Christmas. So, I guess anything can happen.

Back to pizza. It's so easy, it's embarrassing to think I don't do it more.

Mix together 3 cups of your own flours (another solid reason to make your own), a pinch of salt, one cup warm water, and two teaspoons of dried active yeast (one package). That's it! Roll out into a pizza shape, place on cooking surface; pizza stone, whatever (I found the pizza pans full of holes you can find in the grocery store work really well.) Coat with olive oil, Italian seasoning, *your* sauce (you'll be making your own too, if you don't already, it's so much better). Or just pile on veggies, whatever you like. I try to keep a good chunk of feta cheese and spinach in the freezer for my pizzas but you can top it with anything you want. Cook for about 20 min.

Note: Our young missionary friends said they love pizza so we made this recipe together the days they came to help us build our house as their service project.

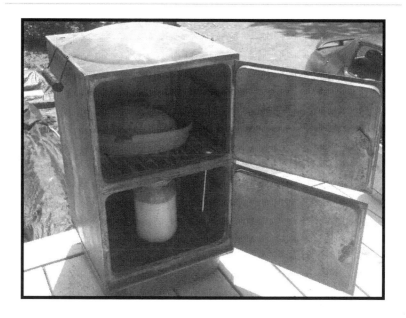

12. WWGD?
(WHAT WOULD GRANDMA DO?)
December 12, 2013

I am planning to make a stew in my grandmother's Griswold number nine cast iron kettle and treasured top that fits it and I think that anything new I need right now to make dinner and feather the nest of our home had better be pretty old if it is going to be of any use. In the last few years as Mike and I have been transitioning out of the rat race to the slow pace, we have been acquiring much needed knowledge and gear. Some of it, like the compact solar power system we are developing for ourselves are not old but the idea of employing all of the benefits of the sun while considering house location, light, and heat are not new.

Our grandparents knew how to do things that we need to learn. The beauty of it is in the combined heritage my husband and I bring to the table. It is simple math: with both sets on each side, that is eight people who had something important to teach us and if you add all of their parents and grandparents to the mix and go on down the line, the number of people who have something to teach us, the number grows exponentially.

Sometimes in our haste to try the "New and Improved" that is blasted in our faces 24-7, we forget the powerful quiet of the tried and true. The wonderful technology of the hand-ground polish of an old cast iron pan outlasts any new pan that comes in a glossy box with special instructions. There are no special cleaning powders that come with a cast iron pan; you aren't supposed to clean it much anyway. The best way to keep it clean is to use it for everything. There are no damaging chips of something drummed up in a lab that end up in your body if you use the wrong spoon to stir. Cast iron likes to be heated up empty and scraped clean with a metal spatula or even a balled up piece of tin foil. Admittedly, the pan does leech residue: iron. I am pretty sure my body knows what to do with that.

When deciding what to learn, keep, and what to give away, the test is to be able to answer a few questions: first, can it fill out a form in triplicate to explain when and why we might use it? (It must serve a minimum of three functions.) Second, will it work without electricity and special care? And third, is it something our grandparents would have used or done?

This is how we ended up learning how to grow, can, bee keep, knit, make pots, soap, and preserve food in numerous ways, clear land, set up firewood, and build our own house. I am now learning how to cook on a wood stove. Don't get me wrong, I still have a pretty fancy gas stove in my kitchen but the wood stove serves many purposes at once and uses fuel that we gathered ourselves. In short, it saves us money, and that is something our grandparents were all about.

One of the things I plan to try out today is the Conservo that we found on the internet after visiting a wood stove doctor in Little Compton, Rhode Island. In our journey of examining all wood stove possibilities, Mike and I visited Jim, a retired science teacher and his son who run an expansive business of refurbishing anything and everything that heats and cooks with wood. Their place is a museum of everything Nineteenth Century Americana. The amazing thing is that even the rusty rubble of 150 year old parts piled up on a wooden pallet that he showed us, still had a working door latch. It needed a little work, he told us, but was within our price range. We actually considered it but didn't think we'd have the time to work on it since we had a house to save for and build at that time.

Our new appliances don't even last 15 years before they need to be replaced. Most of them are not made in our country anymore either. American ingenuity and American-made used to mean something that would stand up. I believe it still does, but it is being done in small companies that respond to basic needs with integrity, the same way it started.

While Jim showed us around his warehouses, he pointed out odd little items that were used during the late 1800's and early 1900's when few people had electricity. "This is a great waffle iron you use directly on the wood stove, it sits in a number seven hole," he said as he pawed through items on a disheveled shelf of cast iron, enamel, and galvanized gadgets.

"What's that?" I asked, pointing to a tall rectangular tin box with two small doors attached.

"Oh, that. This is a very special little item. It's hard to find them now. Ours even has the original instruction manual. This is from 1906, it's called a Conservo and it's a steam oven that sits on top of your wood stove. Pretty fancy stuff."

"You see this," he pointed to an odd little pipe sticking out of the top right hand corner of the box, "this sits in a chamber of water that surrounds the oven and whistles when you need to add more water. It works with steam to cook and makes a wonderful baked chicken. You can also can in it without filling your house up with steam."

That began the Conservo adventure. As much as we loved the idea of restoring Jim's rusted collection of parts to make our own Glenwood original wood stove, it wasn't a practical solution to our heating and cooking needs. So we went with a high-efficiency contemporary model that has a catalytic combustion that burns the creosote right out of the pine (a plus when you consider how precious our wood is and that a good portion of our wood is pine). But the Conservo was a different story. We couldn't offer Jim enough to part with his Conservo, so we searched on line and found a reasonable one that needed a little care.

I am not sure if either of our sets of grandparents owned a Conservo; there weren't too many made and they cost $12.00 during the Depression years. Our grandparents may have considered it an expensive luxury gadget. But we are happy to add it to our wood stove since it can answer our other two questions with alacrity: yes, it performs more than three functions, and yes, it can be used without electricity and special care. It's a keeper. If Grandma could taste her chicken recipe made in the Conservo, I think she would be pleased with our family's progress.

MAKING YOGHURT

I have found that most things that need to proof or set up must be kept between 90 and 110 degrees (body temperature).

Even if you can't get whole, unpasteurized milk where you live, you can still make your own yoghurt. I have been doing it for years and I shudder to think how many of those 16 ounce plastic containers I would have accumulated over that time span. For that alone, I think it's worth it. I used to use a handy electric yoghurt maker that cost about $40 or so. It's worth it. I repurposed the silly little jars they provide you with and got a glass container with a rubber lid that fit the machine and used that instead. The lid keeps it nice and fresh in the fridge when your yoghurt is done.

If you are an exacting type, my recipes probably drive you crazy. In that case you have already ordered the electric appliance and will go by its instruction manual. If you're like me and can make a meal from the crumbs you find in the couch cushions, this recipe is for you.

Take any amount of milk you have on hand. Use up the old stuff first. Whole milk makes the best yoghurt. Heat it up as slowly as you have time for. Turn it off when it starts to look like it will boil over. You can still use it if it does boil over, it's just a mess you'll have to clean up right away and who has time for that? Yoghurt experts say the film on top of the milk will inhibit the culture. I never noticed the difference. I'm not an expert on yoghurt but I am expert at letting things boil-over so I used to set my timer for 13 minutes to keep the boil-over from happening once again. Then let it cool. You can put it in a sink of cool water if you want to speed things up. It should cool until it reaches between 90 and 110 degrees. Since that's body temperature, if you can hold your finger in it for any length of time, it's ready.

Add a few good dollops (okay, about a ½ cup or so) of

a good yoghurt as a starter. You can also buy a pricey powder starter in your health food store. Eventually, you'll use your own yoghurt as a starter (just always save a dollop of it in the jar). Greek yoghurt has different cultures so if you like it, use it as a starter. If you have to use whole milk from your grocery store, add a few tablespoons of dried milk for a thicker consistency.

I use a stoneware jar with a lid in the winter to make mine. Depending on how hot the wood stove, I either put it on the warming trivet on the back of the stove or in my Conservo right next to the stove. It sets up right away. It must be kept between 90-110 degrees to set. Rule of thumb, if the proofing area is too hot to touch, it is not body temperature.

In the summer, I place the warmed milk and yoghurt in a Mason jar and proof it on the deck in my Conservo. A simple oven thermometer is a helpful device to keep track of the temperature.

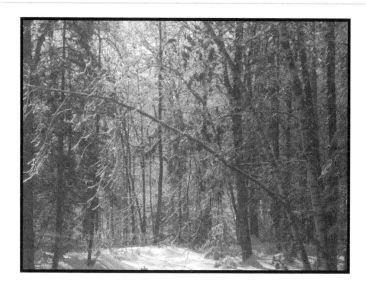

13 BEAUTY
December 21, 2013

Whenever we are asked how we ended up this far north, Mike and I usually say that we fell in love with the beauty of the wilderness.

Most writers have found ways to describe the beauty they see and feel. Many delve into the terrible beauty of human nature, that intricate labyrinth of light and shadow that motivates our actions. Many, like painters and photographers, choose to re-create the landscapes they find in their search. Though some are successful, they must admit that a re-creation is just that. Their works will always pale when compared to the real thing.

Like Thoreau and Emerson, the only thing my words can possibly attempt to do is describe how the beauty I see around me affects my interior nature. The majesty of witnessing a bald eagle fly overhead while you play in the waters of a pristine river is impossible to duplicate with words. I can only try to relate to you the transformation it has made in me. To find the true beauty of a moment such as this, you must experience it yourself. Ultimately, beauty is such a personal process.

As I watch the river freeze up and the snow fall in recognizable flakes creating a glittering finish on the undercoat of a blue-white snow, I think I understand why white is the universal color of purity. Nature has deemed it so as she eliminates our human litter from the landscape and reclaims her own. Every bit of the inevitable clutter of human sin is erased in one cool sweep of her wand. My eyes receive a much-needed rest from my to-do list, as everything I should have picked up and organized disappears from view. My nerves are calm as I focus on the task of staying warm and fed. I call it the Bilbo Baggins lifestyle of warm milk and sweet biscuits. It becomes essential to my health as my body calls for the rest.

When I discover that I have used up the batteries in my radio, I am reduced to a humble symphony of silence that is not silent at all. I listen to the power of the river, even as it is half-frozen. I hear a hawk's singular song and spy a flock of wild turkey crossing through the forest. They appear glad that Mike plowed since they can use the driveway as respite from their lumbered half-flight through the thickening snow and jostle from rock to bent tree in their search for food.

When we notice the tracks of a larger-than-housecat feline, probable a lynx, we notice how it follows the road. The animals like it that we create roads. The deer and moose move more easily through them, conserving much-needed calories when the snow covers their food. Perhaps our being here is not so aberrant, I think.

"The snow cover is hard on the deer," our friend Richard tells us when we work with him on a construction job. "Many of them just starve to death."

Richard explained to me that he spends close to two thousand dollars a year to feed the deer. He showed me a picture of over a hundred gathered in his yard to feed. It's impressive.

When I asked him about hunting them, he said he doesn't anymore. "They fed my boys as I raised them. Now it's my turn to give back."

I knew he really meant it when he said they fed his boys because after his wife left him, Richard raised his family of three boys by himself. I think he understands a little bit about going hungry in the winter.

Winter around here is no joke. A few nights ago the temperatures went down to minus 27. It takes just a few minutes outside without gloves to know what that means to a person's ability to survive. It is hard to stay warm when the body has no fuel, no matter how many layers of wool you pack on. If processed with respect, one deer will provide enough fat and protein for a person to live on for an entire year.

Richard tells me that the deer can't digest certain grains like corn. Even the oats he feeds them requires at least six weeks before their digestive tracks obtain enough of the enzyme they need to process the starches. He is well-aware that the deer become dependent upon him in the winter as their digestive chemistry changes; they can't metabolize their natural fare anymore, until they go through another adjustment period. He's okay with that since the deer population has been on a steady decline and most of the deer that visit him would probably have starved to death.

I consider offering the deer the five gallon bucket of acorns I collected but I think again. It would be a foolish endeavor. We have to focus on us first. Richard is a grandfather now with a successful construction business he runs with his sons. He has provided well for his family. Someday I will be able to give back too but today is not the day.

In spite of what most people may think, hunting is beautiful. First, statistically speaking, only 14% of deer hunters actually take down a deer. It's not that easy. Deer are really smart and sassy. We stopped to speak to a hunter who had parked on our road consistently for a few weeks. He told us he had not caught a single deer all season but wanted to tell us a funny story.

"So there I was, being so careful to hide my scent and be as stealthy and inconspicuous as possible, quiet, you know, and there he was, the biggest buck I've ever seen right behind me almost staring over my shoulder. I turned ever so slowly to see him but he was just too close, you know. And he just looked at me. Then he took off. Do you know that buck walked right up to me right in my own footsteps. Son of a gun!"

Mike and I have decided that we like sitting in the deer stand together. It's more fun. We don't talk. We communicate through nudges. Mike likes to research everything so one of the latest books he downloaded on his kindle is about deer hunting. We discovered we have been doing a lot wrong. But being out in the forest, completely silent and covered in dirt and leaves is one of the most thrilling things I have ever done.

Having chipmunks and squirrels climb over your legs as though you're not there is cool. You get to see what goes on in the world without human chatter to interrupt. The forest is absolutely beautiful with all of its moss and mini kingdoms of florescent fungi. Creatures of the forest have much to teach us. They play.

One night Mike saw about fifteen deer. He couldn't safely shoot any so he waited and came home with only the story of a curious barn owl to tell. Mike's stories are always funny. I couldn't help but wonder what story a barn owl might tell his wife that night about the clumsy hunter that went through great pains to try and go unnoticed. I could just see him imitating all of the twigs and ferns stuck in this silly hunter's hat and how ridiculous it was to think you could pretend to be a part of something you clearly are not. It takes a lot of time to earn the privilege of catching a buck. It takes reverence, prayer, knowledge, skill, and Mother Nature has to then deem you worthy. In the meantime, it's just plain fun to try.

Like hunting, foraging and beauty go together. When you forage, you notice the beauty. In fact, what I have noticed is that a lot of the things that are edible are beautiful like cattails, milkweed, chicken mushrooms, acorns, all of the berries, the fiddleheads, and the flowers and herbs used for tea. White pine possesses a soft loveliness that other pines don't. Knowing what to look for and what you're looking at reveals the intricacies of nature.

Mike and I plan to take another trip up the Allagash someday soon. Like all pilgrims, we feel we must return to the place of our great awakening, if only to say thank you and to reconnect. Our bodies will be a little softer, our minds, a little quieter, but our spirits are already there.

HUNTING DEER

First let me tell you, I have never taken down a deer so what I am about to tell you is stuff we have learned to try and do next time we go out.

Smell: Deer can smell you and your clothes. Good hunters use no-scent detergent on their hunting clothes and then store them in a bag with cedar chips.

Sight: Deer can see you really well if you go out in jeans. They see blue as ultra-violet. They can't see neon orange. They see you if you are wearing one color, even if it's forest green because they detect your form as a weird shadow. Hence, the camouflage-neon orange gear sold to hunters. Also, the neon orange is required to keep you safe from crossfire. Humans apparently aren't as perceptive as the deer in this respect.

Sound: You have to take a vow of silence if you want to see a deer. Even breathing loud or rustling leaves or branches while you shift about will alert them. If it weren't for the foul odor, I think zombies might be good deer hunters.

Movement: All animals, including humans, detect movement before they pick up any other indicator. Even if you have a red squirrel tickling your nose, you have to stay perfectly still.

Your own comfort: It is key to be able to maintain all of these other items intact that you make yourself a comfortable place to wait and see. If you make a deer blind on the ground, you have to make it in advance or they'll hear you cutting branches and gathering leaves and know immediately you're up to no good. Even if they aren't anywhere near you, all of the other animals will let them know as soon as they pass through the area. We don't have one, but the tree stand is probably a good way to avoid squirrel-crossings. Though, it appears that owls think they're pretty funny, so good luck.

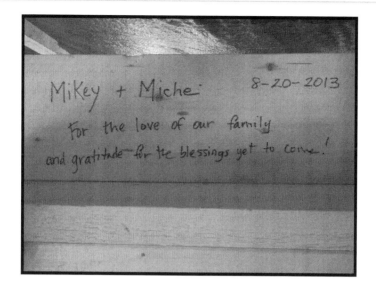

14. LOVE AND FEAR
December 28, 2013

Mike and I have been called a few things by people we know, most of them labels we own up to, like "crazy", "dreamers" - the usual. When people start to mock us for being "preppers" and operating under the assumption that we can insulate ourselves from some future fearful occurrence, we say, "Not so much."

We made our move to a simpler life for the same reason many have done it. We love it. We love being masters of our ship, deciding that we want to go skiing when the weather is good, not when we have our week off from work and are forced to wait in long lift lines. We love being together, no matter what the job, and this lifestyle affords that for us. We love to wake up in the middle of the night and see shooting stars, Northern Lights, and the Milky Way.

The reason for building our lives out here is not fear but love. Love, I have come to understand, is a more powerful motivator than fear. One of the reasons I grew increasingly impatient and discontent with my work as a public school teacher is that schools often try to motivate students through fear more than through love. We threaten students with the fear that if they don't learn whatever it is and score well on a test, they are sliding toward failure. Of course, many students see right through that argument and it holds no power over them. Take the logic behind a commonly used argument in a lot of high school counselors' offices (not all, of course), "if you don't do your homework, study, make the grades, and graduate, you will remain in entry-level jobs the rest of your life." This is just the apex of the mountain of fear-based lies this kid has had to listen to his whole life. His entire being has resisted these lies for years but he has managed to force himself to go back to school year after year. He has wasted his vital energy on all of this conflict inside of him because fear is always **false evidence appearing real**. It's an exhausting occupation for everyone.

Most teachers know that if you took that student ten years ago, got to know him, found out what he loves, and then built your case for education on what he loves, then you have something there. It's not forced, it's nurtured. When his intellect is treated as a living, growing thing that is respected and loved, I believe you will experience a different outcome. He will keep coming back to learning year after year because he loves to learn. It is his birthright.

The term "preppers" implies a certain negativity. They are people who are motivated by the fear that something catastrophic is going to happen and they want to be ready for it. From what I have experienced, fear debilitates. People who are truly fearful never take any action. They get mired in it.

People who believe that our world economy may shift and that their lifestyles may change are just being pragmatic since change is the only constant. In a large and complex economy where even a simple item like a loaf of bread on the family table has been shipped a few times before its first slice is buttered, knowing that food sources will change is being realistic. Perhaps it is more important to know what is in that bread. It might also be wise to break down the personal expense it took to buy that bread. When the above has been considered by a rational person who loves himself, his health, and his family, he may be inspired to go out and purchase some whole grain flour and some bread yeast.

He soon realizes that he loves to make bread. He gets good at it; he shares his bread. He may decide that he would rather make bread than rush off to work in the morning and swing by and pick up a puffed-up loaf at the store before heading home. He begins to experiment with things that go with bread like jams and cheeses. He discovers that cheese is better when made with unpasteurized milk. He begins to find out how homogenizing milk makes it impossible for the body to metabolize its fats. He discovers that pasteurizing milk kills the enzymes the human body needs to digest it. He begins to look for farmers who will sell him raw milk and he discovers that it is illegal in his state to sell it.

This is the journey of just one questioning, loving person who decides to experience life outside the bread box and see what it is like. He discovers that life is a lot richer since he stopped eating sliced bread and homogenized milk. His blood pressure decreases. He's more energetic. He is happier. He desires to do more, love more. He feels more alive. This gives him the energy and courage he needs to make the change he would like to make. His dreams become promises to himself.

It happens just like this. Any dream can come true if a person is willing to do what it takes to make it happen. For Mike and me, our dream was to live off the grid in a cabin in the woods and to write and travel. Dreams cannot be fulfilled with a fearful heart; it is simply not powerful enough. Fostering a dream requires too much to learn. Dreams can only be followed with a loving heart. In fact, nothing will undermine a dream faster than a little bout of fear. One fearful comment from someone else can set a dreamer's timeline back years. It could even destroy the person's ability to believe it possible. Nothing can kill a dream faster than a tiny drop of fear. It's toxic.

Knowing this, why do we try to motivate children with it? For the same reason we will feed them store-bought bread and factory-raised milk. My dream is to not be a part of it, even if it means that if I want a slice of toast, I have to knead my own bread first. Perhaps I will find some students who would like to bake bread with me while reading Whitman and Dickinson. These folks knew something about love. They composed for it, knowing they could never insulate themselves from life's pains, but trusting that there is more to life than fear. Perhaps the unwritten message of all crazy dreamers is that love, in all of its tenderness, is more potent than fear.

FAMILY LOAF

I found an old cast-iron pan that makes twelve little loaf-ettes that are delightful for lunches on the go or with tea. Mike always vies for the heel when I bake a loaf of bread. The loaf-ettes provide him with crusty little heels all week long. I like them because they are a lot less crumby than a loaf and anything that saves me housework is my friend. Mixing in valuable seeds and nuts adds flavor and nutrition. Our family loaf truly is the staff of life.

Take a nice bowl you can hug and put 1 ½ cups warm water, 3 tablespoons of cooking oil, 3 tablespoons of yoghurt, two tablespoons of brown sugar, 1 ½ teaspoons of salt, a couple of handfuls of unsalted mixed nuts and seeds (I keep this on hand for muesli and other recipes – just keep adding seeds and nuts as you pick them up- sunflower, pumpkin, walnuts, sliced almonds, pistachios -what a treat to find a little emerald treasure in your loaf-ette, flax seeds (you get the idea), another couple of handfuls of 10-grain cereal (or whatever whole grain mix you can get- wheat germ is good), and then 4 ¼ cups regular flour. I'm not sure why, but measuring the flour well by spooning it into your measuring cup and taking a knife and clearing off the top is really important for your dough. I think it has to do with adding air to the flour. Also, measure your 2 teaspoons of yeast carefully, making sure it doesn't heap up over the measuring spoon.

Hug your bowl and mix it all with your hand. When it's good and sticky, turn it out onto your countertop with some flour on hand to knead it. The purpose of kneading dough is to get pockets of air all caught up into it so it will rise. Have fun and play with it. Most recipes say allow your dough to rise twice. I never do. I'm just plain impatient. I set my dough into a greased loaf (or loaf-ette) pan and let it rise on the back of the wood stove. When it is double in size, I pop it into a 350 degree oven for 30-35 minutes and well, do I have to tell you what the smell of fresh-baking bread does to a house?

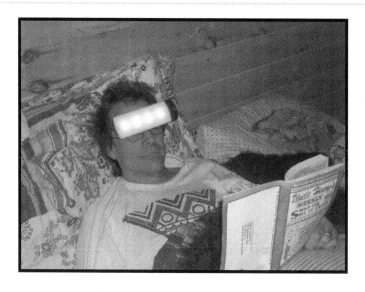

15. A TWELVE STEP PROCESS
December 30, 2013

It is hard to tell if it was the negative ions in the air due to the impending storm or that Mike and I were just plain exhausted, but yesterday was remarkable in its inefficiency. By the time we finally gave up on all of the mishaps of our day and decided to locate our snowshoes and go for a walk, we had expended every ounce of juice we had left in us. We went to bed with the chickens at 4:30. Fortunately, we had charged the solar batteries up so we could both use our lamps. I like the bedroom lamps because they produce a warm golden light that neither jars nor strains. It is the antidote for the heavy darkness that can set into a soul this time of year.

To appreciate the quality of our day yesterday, I must first explain that Mike and I pushed ourselves to drive to Bangor to pick up the black iron pipe we would need to install the gas lamps in the kitchen and bathroom and streamline the gas hook-ups for the stove and refrigerator. We were intent on beating a storm and getting all of the supplies we would need to settle in and get some work done on the house since we wouldn't be able to get to the construction job we were both working on for a few days. The first indication that our get-ahead-fast plan might not be a smooth road was that our car began to sputter and choke at indeterminate intervals on our way to town. Being forty minutes from the nearest friend and the temperature hovering at around zero, we were a bit nervous. Luckily, our car, "Sherman" (named after the tank), got us there and back and Mike seems to think he knows what the problem is. Nevertheless, we are aware that Mike needs to perform a check-up and repair before we travel too much and too far again.

Since it was already pretty late when we got back home, we left the iron pipe in the car. What we experienced the next morning was a perfect example of how the twelve-step process is the inevitable result of the two-step process. The first thing Mike wanted to get done yesterday was that easy two-step process of plowing the driveway. Brush off truck and plow. He would be done by 8:30, he told me. Not quite: after exclaiming, "Hey, why is the rear wheel locking up?" we figured it might take a little longer to plow.

Then we were going to retrieve some equipment from the carport/ storage shed when we discovered that it had collapsed from the weight of the snow: *"When did that happen!!!?"* I wiggled in and rescued the plastic bin of family photos I had forgotten to store in the house earlier. Everything else will have to wait until spring if we need it. One of the items I had been searching for is the small kitchen scale I needed in order to make soap. (Fortunately, I found two bars in amongst other stuff in the basement. That should hold us over until I can figure it out. But that is another twelve-step story).

"Go ahead and take a shower," Mike told me. He had managed to set the tile in the shower floor the day before and was going to grout it and tile the sides of the shower that day. He assured me that it would dry without any issues if I showered early. I was happy to oblige.

The propane hot water heater that he had researched and purchased on line works so well that I have to temper it with the cold water to get it just right. After some months of using a tub of water heated on the wood stove, hot showers still feel like a treat to me. Wanting to be sure that we possess full control over our hot water and not wanting to waste any of it, we installed a manual mixing valve instead of the all-in-one mixing valve that are most common today. It works very well. Except, of course, when the propane tank runs out.

"Honey, I think we are out of propane. My shower just turned cold."

"Hang on, I'll just move the tank from the stove to the hot water heater in the basement. It will take just a second."

I tried to stay put so that his efforts wouldn't be wasted, but got cold and decided that a hot, steamy shower just wasn't in the cards. I also figured that the less water I used in the shower, the faster it would dry up and be ready for Mike's tile work.

Mike had come in from "plowing" to tell me that the truck kept getting stuck in reverse so before he could plow, he would have to take the rear wheels off and see what was causing the trouble. I helped him find his insulated coveralls, a good pair of mechanic's gloves, and a good dose of warm appreciation since it was below zero. The two-step process of dusting off the truck and getting in it to plow had now turned into a several step process, including digging it out enough to get to the back tires. Gathering and finding tools that have multi-uses adds more steps to the process.

My attempts at making soap had been thwarted early on by the discovery of the shed disaster so I decided to make bread instead. By noontime, Mike managed to get the truck unstuck, claiming it was a miracle. He came in, ate some baked beans and warm bread and decided to get started on the shower.

"The shower is still wet." I popped my head in and could see that the tiles had not fully set when I took my "shower" that morning and everything was still damp in the bathroom. "I will put the small propane heater in here and try to dry it out," he said. That, of course, required that he take the tank off of the hot water heater in the basement and hook it up to the small space heater in the bathroom. "Hey, when did this thing stop working?"

After another half hour, he got the heater to work. "I'm not going to be able to work on the tile today. It needs to dry out some more before I can grout it. Let me see about installing the black pipe instead so we can eliminate all of these propane tanks."

That's when he discovered that one of the black pipes must have slid forward on the console of the car and caused a crack in the windshield.

"We are going to have to take Sherman in to replace his windshield too," Mike said, hanging his head in the resignation that springs out of the deep well of his inimitable good nature. It had been a day of just too many steps and he was willing to simply surrender to a power much greater than his own.

"Maybe we ought to just eat some cookies, drink some milk, and then go for a walk." I had already taken care of steps one and two in this little plan, but I still had to put on my coat, boots, and gloves to dig around in the snow for the snow shoes I had stored under the camper in September. Fortunately, they were exactly where I thought they would be and I didn't have to dig at all. Mike wasn't sure it was worth the effort but I insisted.

"Let's get out and play a little. It is so beautiful out there." When I appeared with snow shoes and poles in hand a few minutes later, Mike agreed that it would be good for us. I ran up the ladder to the loft and grabbed a couple of the hand warmers we gave ourselves for Christmas just in case. He put on the ski pants I had put aside earlier and we strapped on our snow shoes.

"We're going to have to plow tomorrow," Mike says. That goes for every other project we started today.

A REAL SOAP OPERA

I have noticed that my intros to these how-to's are a lot longer than the recipes. The truth is, it takes time to make your own stuff. You have to have a darned good reason to want to do it. Take soap, for instance. You can buy it anywhere. It's cheap. It gets you clean. What's the problem?

The problem is that what you are purchasing is detergent, not soap. Detergent strips whatever it washes of its oils. It's great for dishes but, not for skin or hair. Soap contains fats that dissolve the dirt that binds to our oils but it doesn't strip all of the oil out of our skin. We need these natural oils to protect our skin.

You can get hand-milled, Castile, or glycerin soap in most health-food markets but they can be pricey. When you start using them, you will realize how much damage most store-bought stuff does to your skin. I like to think of my skin as my most important organ. Its job is to protect me and my other precious organs. The job of my brain (another important organ) is to protect my skin.

Once we started using our own soap, we tried making a shampoo bar. Since then, we have never gone back to the bottle. Then we made our own shaving soap and kicked the can. In fact, we have kicked the entire personal-care-isle addiction right out of our lives.

I no longer battle winter rosacea and where to store the myriad bottles of special conditioners that I once used to tame my frizzy hair. My hair is no longer a huge puff ball since I stopped using shampoo. It wasn't my hair that was the trouble, it was the laurel sulfate!

Okay, enough drama! The recipes, please.

Soap
298 grams coconut oil
298 grams olive oil
255 grams Shea butter
227 grams water
119 grams lye
20 drops essential oil

Shampoo Bar
510 gms olive oil
340 gms palm oil
255 gms water
116 gms lye
20 drops essential oil

There are plenty of U-tube videos and on-line sites to help you with making soap. This is just a brief outline of how it's done. I hope you get the idea that it's not that hard. The main tool you will need is a very good, stainless steel hand mixer. You will burn out the plastic kind really fast, so don't. It's worth it to get a good one. You also need to find lye. Some hardware stores still carry it. It's in the plumbing section because it's used to clear out pipes. This might be the hardest part of the process.

Warm your harder oils together by putting a stainless bowl over a pot of boiling water. If you use good oils, you don't want to ruin them by burning out their great properties, you just need to liquefy them. Keep your oils between 90-110 degrees (body temp range again!) but still liquid.

While this is happening, you can mix the lye and water. Do this outside; it creates caustic fumes that will burn your eyes and all other soft tissue. It will heat up. When it gets to between 90-110 degrees it is ready to use. (Is anybody else seeing a pattern here? – but **don't stick your finger in it to check the temp**- don't touch it!- if it gets on you, wash with kitchen soap and water.)

When everything is ready, add the olive oil to the oils you were melting and then add the lye mixture. Your essential oils go in last or they will dissipate right away and it's a waste. Time to SOPONIFY!!!!

Use the hand blender to mix, trying not to aerate. When it looks like vanilla pudding, add the scent.

Pour into your mold (a paper milk carton will work). **At this phase it is still very caustic – don't touch it.** If you make a reusable mold, make sure you line it with wax paper.

Let it set (it will warm up as it does this). When it is finally room temp you can touch it. Unmold it and cut into bars. Let it sit for some weeks in a basket to ventilate. It will harden and last longer if you do. Curing it this way neutralizes the pH to 7 which is important.

Make sure you sing in the shower when you use your own soap! *Who's the Diva now?*

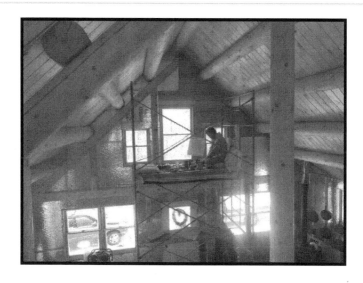

16. TAKING MY TIME
January 1, 2014

Yesterday Mike went into town to work so I decided to surprise him with a special dinner when he got home to celebrate the New Year. I made an Indian style fare using the pumpkin and chick peas I had canned and stored and added a can of coconut milk. I made a pumpkin and ginger soup. I decided to make *naan*, an Indian flat bread in my grandmother's cast iron pan on the stove top. Since it was too cold to get the generator to work in the morning, I would not be able to use the oven on my stove to make a yeast bread. It is a gas stove but the oven needs a small amount of power to operate. With no generator, I ran out of water since the water pump also needs a little power to prime. The larger water tank usually lasts us a day or two and needs to be run for about two minutes to prime again.

We had just picked up our gallon of raw milk from our farmer the day before and we had been so busy the week before that we still had almost a full gallon in the fridge. I decided to make Mike's favorite dessert, tapioca pudding, and a queso blanco (simple white cheese) with the milk. Mike loves the whey which is the byproduct of making cheese. I mixed it with a little honey and some nutmeg to make a healthier alternative to eggnog. Whey is delicious and is a good source of protein without any fat.

Since we still have Larry's scaffolding up on the gable end of the house to finish installing the tongue and groove paneling, I decided that it would be fun to set our table up in the air, by the three front windows, overlooking the stars. I thought that one of the pleasures of having a little party is the morning after when you get to pick at the leftovers so I would set out dried fruits and nuts, sliced oranges, the cheese, and enough food for the morning. Sitting up high, overlooking the river, would be a nice way to start our New Year.

I brought up some candles and fashioned a mood lamp out of a white shade I made and the LED Christmas tree lights I took off the tree. Some nice linens, silverware, pretty glasses for the whey and water, and the surprise was complete.

Between carting all of the components of our fancy dinner up a double set of scaffolding and cooking everything from scratch, including a batch of yoghurt, I didn't accomplish much else that day. Once everything was set, I put on a nice silk top and practiced a little yoga while I awaited Mike's arrival.

Since our table was set about fifteen feet up in the cathedral ceiling, Mike didn't notice it when he got home. He could tell something was up, though. I said something silly to him like, "Hey, you want to get high with me?" to which he smirked. He asked if I would like to go into town since he didn't see any dinner activity. I said, no, I just wanted to have a little fun with him. That's when he noticed the mood lamp and gave me a querulous look. I smiled and said, "Follow me."

Seeing the look of wonder and pleasure on my husband's face made all of my preparations worthwhile. I knew I would enjoy the Indian-inspired feast, but knowing that I could fully share that joy with my husband made it all complete.

Being able to take my time and carry each item up one at a time during the day made the entire day memorable and the fare that much more beautiful. Being relaxed and calm when Mike got home set the tone for a pleasant evening.

Thinking it might be a nice activity, I set out a little wooden platter with two strips of paper and a pen to write out any notes to self for the New Year. I originally thought I might write down things I would like to **stop** doing and Mike said that he was writing things he **will** do instead. I agreed. That is a much better approach to life and I decided to do the same.

We took our time writing the notes and discussing our goals for the year. We talked about our relationship, our accomplishments, our girls, and things we enjoy doing together. We took care to write things we are sure we want to do because there's one thing about Mike and me, if we say we are going to do something, we do it. I got excited for the year ahead, thinking about our plans.

My list included making sure that I fully embrace my life and the people in it. That would mean no room for doubts or reservations about the future and following my dreams. It means a lot more hugging. Mike said he wanted to fish more. I agreed that was a good one. We each wrote a few more things that were meaningful to us. Then I wrote, "Take my time."

Just thinking about this made me tear up. Raising two girls while working full-time and trying my hardest to make sure they had what they needed, to grow to be strong and capable had meant constant multi-tasking and urgent activity. Most mothers will agree this becomes the modus operandi until the kids are out on their own. I heartily applaud those who are able to take their time to slow down and enjoy life while raising children. If I could do it all again, I would take my time. But I can't undo life so I have to just undo the way I live the rest of it. This is not such an easy task when you have so much practice doing it the other way through most of it.

So, I made it a New Year's affirmation and am working on it becoming my new MO. It starts with taking my time to breathe. The other end of the spectrum is resolving to slow down as I write and plan my next move. There will be plenty of time to align all of the small tasks involved in working again and trying to publish. I will take my time, I have decided.

Everything else will fall into place.

Mike was glad that he did not have to rush out and find an open place to eat on New Year's Eve. The temperature was twenty-something below zero and the two restaurants in town were probably both closed. He had worked hard that day in our friend's auto shop. What he needed most was to come home to a warm house, a hot shower, and a wife who had taken her time making a memorable meal.

Affirmative.

INDIAN FLAT BREAD

This bread can be made with any mixture of whole grain and nut flours. It is a versatile, fast bread that can serve as a respite from gluten and yeast. We used to eat it in Trinidad where I spent some of my formative years.

Mix 2 cups flour, ½ teaspoon baking soda, pinch of salt, ¾ cup yoghurt, 1 tablespoon melted butter, oil for pan cooking.

The dough should mix up firmly. Roll into a ball, leave in mixing bowl, and cover with a cloth for fifteen minutes. Pinch off enough dough to make 2 inch balls. Roll them out until they are 1/8 inch thick and brush over with a little melted butter on both sides. Use a cast iron pan to griddle them since it can heat up nicely and you'll use less oil.

Best if served warm. We keep ours on a warming trivet on the back of our wood stove.

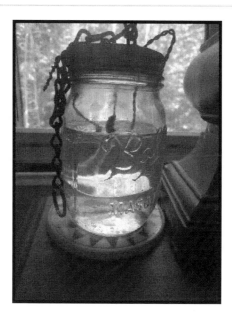

17. STARS
January 14, 2014

Just about every Mainer you run into asks if you've been up here any length of time in the winter. In fact, you'd have to say that *Mainiacs* are completely obsessed by the weather. According to the folks in these parts, there are four seasons in Maine: Snow, Mud, Black Fly, and Construction. In most cases, they all pretty much run together. It has been known to snow in July up here. And as for Black Flies, well it's an experience everyone should have at least once in life. Let's just say, it's humbling.

As I ice skated my way across the six feet from my car to my friend's front porch last night, I was reminded why the obsession. I also understand why Mainers seem to have a lot of stuff in their yards. Fortunately, in mid-November we decided to take advantage of some tire sales and put new snow tires with studs on our car. We changed the back tires on Mike's work van and bought chains for the plow truck. With everything iced over the way it has been for the past two weeks, the only vehicle we have been able to use is the car with four-wheel drive and studded snow tires. The work van just skids around and ends up crooked in the snow banks any time Mike tries to get it going.

In order to walk anywhere in our driveway and yard, I have to attach a pair of metal cleats to my thick rubber boots or I will end up sliding in all directions. It is not very comfortable to lose control of your feet when you walk.

Weather in Maine will force a slow-down.

Living with no electrical hook-up in the winter up here is, well, let's not sugar-coat-it, dark. Darkness, I have discovered, is not modern man (or woman's) best friend.

Humanity has struggled much just so that it can turn on a light switch when the world outside gets dark. Around the winter equinox, sunset happens slightly shy of four o'clock. Out here, darkness can feel a little intimidating. To combat the negative effects of the darkness, Mike installed a propane gas lamp in the kitchen and, lacking solar power, we use a small inverter to run two bedside lamps to read by at night. We use two LED light bulbs in our lamps that give off a soft golden light at night. So far, it works out fine, even though we are usually in bed by 6:30 on those winter nights.

The up-side to the darkness is the reality that it usually isn't all that dark. In fact, winter nights are frequently so crisp that in the battle between stars and snowflakes, the snowflakes are vastly outnumbered. Some nights up here, I feel as though I have the time to sit still and count to be sure. I spent the first fifty years of my life wondering what the elusive Milky Way really looks like. Up here, I see it just about every night. The only way to see it is to have an unadulterated view of the night sky. That means, no light pollution.

About twenty-five years ago, I caught a segment on National Public Radio about this group of people in New Hampshire who were trying to pass legislation on outdoor lighting. Their aim was not to eliminate it, but to shield the lights so that they illuminated only downward toward the street, yard, or parking lot. I always thought this was a noble idea. Light pollution robs us of our place in the universe and makes us uneasy in the dark.

A friend recently wrote that when we teach our children about the constellations, they see the starry night sky as a familiar story-book populated with characters and their adventures. When children learn how and when to search out these characters, they never feel quite alone under the night sky. Darkness is no longer a place of uncertainty and fear. It is a place of discovery and wonder.

I agree. Everyone has a favorite constellation, I am learning. Most people in our hemisphere locate the Big Dipper, Ursa Major, who is up there with her son Ursa Minor (Little Dipper). Ursa comes from the word Bear so Mamma Bear and Baby Bear are up there together. In one telling of the story, Mamma and Baby Bear keep each other company in the heavens. If you follow the top of Ursa Major (the top of the Dipper) over about four times the distance of the two top stars, you will locate the North Star. This is a good thing to know.

My favorite is Orion. He is the hunter with a bow in one hand, a scabbard hanging from his belt (one of those stars is Betelgeuse), and an arrow pointing right at the bull (Taurus). Orion is protecting the Seven Sisters (the Pleiades) from the bull. Orion also has a buddy who helps him. You can see this friend under his left foot in the winter but you have to wait until Orion has risen a bit. This is man's best friend: Sirius.

The sky tells me this story year after year and I never tire of it. In fact, I look forward to winter, just so I can say hello to my friends again. Beyond the familiar story of rescue and loyalty is the personal symbolism I always derive from Orion. There he is, eternally holding the wild, brutish forces at bay so that the seven sisters can cluster together, arguably their greatest asset.

I look to Orion as a symbol of the warrior spirit in me. At a time when darkness rules and the limbic regions of our brains obsess about weather and our ability to stay warm and well-fed, Orion shows up to say, "Don't worry, I got this!" He never actually has to shoot the bull. His posture says it all: "Don't even try it because I am aimed and ready." All I have to do on a night when I am awakened by nervousness or doubt, is to gaze through my bedroom window, and there he is, during the darkest time of the year when I need it most, winking at me.

So when my friend asks me about how I am dealing with the harsh weather and the darkness, I smile and say, "It is pretty dark, that's true, but you should see the stars this time of year!"

A RELIABLY SAFE OIL LAMP

Materials: mason jar and ring (any clear, heat resistant container will do also), any liquid cooking oil, a strand of 100% cotton string or mop (the wick), flexible wire, a common screw driver, optional pieces of small chain for hanging.

How to: wrap the wire around the screw driver until you have formed a ¼ inch long tube and feed the wick through the tube. Use the remaining wire to form a hook to hang the wick from the top of the jar. (Some use a three-wire system so the wick stays put in the middle of the jar.) Add a few tablespoons of oil to the jar, saturating the wick as you do so. Add the water last. The water should bring the oil up to the level of the wick. Lighting the wick takes a little longer since cooking oil burns more slowly. Trim the wick each time you relight it.

Benefits: Other than being a handy idea, this lamp burns so cool that you can safely use it in a tent. If it tumbles, it puts itself out, and because of the water, it illumines in all directions, more like a bulb than a candle.

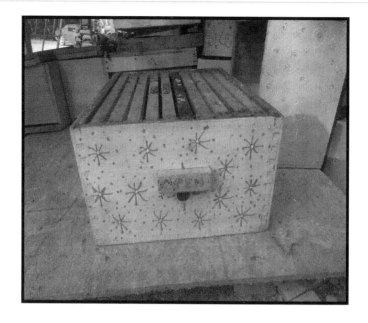

18. MINDING MY OWN BEESWAX
February 3, 2014

As conflictual as it sounds, I always tell people who ask, that beekeeping is a lesson in disappointment that provides unequal levels of satisfaction. It's not an occupation for the faint of heart but is good for such a malady. The simple act of sitting next to a hive on a sunny day and watching the worker bees fly in and out will lull you into a peaceful harmony by their hum. It is probably as close to Nirvana as any Buddhist will get. It produces in me a tranquility that can only come from a higher source. For that experience alone, I would be a beekeeper.

If there needed to be any other reason than a sense of peaceful harmony with Mother Nature and the Great Mind that created such magic, there is the fact that honey bees are nature's most excellent alchemists. They gather nectar from just about everything beautiful and optimize their surroundings to create liquid gold. They are meticulous housekeepers, organizing and cleaning the hive constantly, discarding anything that no longer serves them.

As I observe our bees, I think I will try to be more like them and I believe we do have a lot in common. For one thing, when I feel cold and need to bundle up, they are clustering and staying warm, keeping the surrounding area of the hive at the exact same temperature as a healthy human body. As winter sets in and I feel slower and less willing to brave the outdoors, our bees are doing the same. But, if there's a nice sunny day in winter and the temperature rises to the upper twenties and thirties, the bees will take cleansing flights. I did much the same thing today, taking a walk around the surrounding forest with Hermes to get some fresh air and see what kind of animal tracks I can spot.

While staying indoors where I am warm and drinking a cup of tea is a nice choice, there are days when I need to shake off the luxury, get a little cold and uncomfortable and clear out my head. It is wonderful. But then I discovered how many bees got stuck in the snow on their morning cleansing flights - a fatal error. I wanted to rescue them but they were already frozen. It is sad but it happens.

Bees produce a natural caulking material to seal up their boxes for the winter. It is an orangey-brown glue called propolis and it takes a good bit of leverage to loosen its grip. That's why Mike and I like to mix up some concentrated protein patties for them and place them on the hive before the first frost. The only time you want to break that seal is when you check on them in the spring. It's far better to just put your ear up next to the hive and listen for the hum. Otherwise, it's best just to leave them to their business during the winter. Some beekeepers wrap their hives up in tar paper, leaving a few openings for air flow and cleansing fliers. Every year we claim we are going to get around to it and then don't. Our bees seem to be okay when left to their own devices.

I guess that's true of just about all of us. I find myself worrying unnecessarily about my daughters sometimes. I find myself worrying about my parents and whether I have disappointed them. It sounds silly but I bet a lot of us worry about being disappointed and disappointing the ones we love.

And yet, having kids and being a part of a family is one of the most satisfying enterprises of the human experience. There you have it. Just like the bees. There's always a risk when you get that close to Nirvana. And, so there are times when you make fatal mistakes that cost you a hive or there are times when you did as much as you could possibly do, and you lose the hive anyway.

One thing you will hear experienced beekeepers tell you is, it's a little riskier if you're going to start off with just one hive. In fact, having a few hives makes it more likely you won't lose any. This is mostly true, I guess. But with beekeeping, as with life, there are no guarantees.

My husband makes our bee boxes and I like to paint them in bright colors. The way a bee sees the world is not the way we see it. For one thing, they see white as a fluorescent violet color, almost the effect of using a black light. Nature's beauty is strikingly more attractive for bees. Most wooden bee boxes are painted white. I like to think that adding color to my boxes makes me more cheerful as I approach them and I think the bees like that. I think my bees also like living in such a cool neighborhood of pastel colors and design, less like a cement jungle and more like a garden. It's a fool's game but I think color is important so I leave it at that.

Most people have heard about the vanishing bees. What the bees know is that number one: you can't go around just using Mother Nature like she's an overtime factory worker who desperately needs her job because she's got a mortgage and hungry kids at home. Shipping large quantities of bees all around the country and forcing them to forage all year long is just wrong. It's especially egregious when you give them only one food source and it's contaminated with toxins that jumble their nervous systems and confuse their sense of direction so they can't make it home. Number two: Force-feeding large numbers of hives with corn syrup so they can produce "honey" does not produce honey. It produces processed corn syrup and weak bees. Huge monocultures, chemical additives, and messing with genes by forcing the mass creation of queens is a recipe for disaster and well, the bees know that.

Backyard beekeeping is our way of cuddling up with Mother Nature, giving her the kiss she deserves and letting her bees be. For our own sense of well-being, Mike and I chose to live far enough away from large farms and close to a pure water source and forest cover. Our bees will forage on natural wildflowers and berries this spring. Because we knew we would have to move them, we left them their full supply of honey this winter and are glad we did. It has been a particularly cold winter and they have needed their food supply. Like us, they enjoyed a bountiful fall and took the pains to set themselves up nicely to be warm and well-fed for the winter.

Mike and I have been keeping bees for about seven years now. We still consider ourselves rookies. We started out by signing up for classes at the local university and ordering one complete starter set with the boxes and frames, a feeder, one bee suit, a smoker, and two hive tools. When the time was right in the spring, we visited our local beekeeper who sold us a nuc (a nucleus is a set of worker bees and a live queen). Mike insisted he didn't need a bee suit but a couple of weeks into our little experiment, we ordered the second suit. Beekeeping requires some money up front, there's no doubt. But most beekeepers are frugal sorts and end up making most of their own equipment as they grow.

We lost our hive our first winter. The next year, we ordered two more hives. One of those survived. We added two more the following year and they all survived for the next two years. Each year we added and lost but overall, we experienced a net gain. Two years ago we started out with three hives and ended the summer with eight because of swarming. We learned quickly how to capture a swarm from a nearby tree. We also responded to a call from a contractor to remove bees from a wall in a house he was remodeling. That put us at a total of nine hives. A combination of rookie mistakes and nature's way of keeping hives sustainable left us with four hives at the end of the following winter.

What we gained from all of this experience is a healthy respect for nature and her lovely creatures. We also got shelves full of real, honest-to-goodness honey for ourselves, our family members, and for occasional trading. Now that we have settled in Maine and a simpler lifestyle, we will be studying our hives more closely to create splits and foster queens. We are hoping that the next seven years we will be able to help many people in our area set up their own hives.

We will all be novices, true. But the bees won't be. What I have learned mostly from my bees is analogous to what I have learned about my family and friends. Give the people you love what they need but don't overdo it. Delight in the magic of their beauty but don't let yourself be fooled into thinking you have any control over their destinies. If you can savor the sweetness when it comes your way without taking too much, you'll get the most satisfaction. The best thing, I learned, is to keep up with my own housekeeping. I try to maintain a clean and sunny spot for both my bees and my loved-ones, eliminating the clutter. For the bees that means clearing out old frames and waxy scrapings as that attracts unwanted critters and robbers. In short, minding my own beeswax is the best thing I can do for my bees. That goes for family members too.

LIP ARMOR

This might be the best lip balm you have ever tried. We might as well have called it *Lip Bomb* because it is so high impact. If you check out the ingredients, you'll know why. Nevertheless, our recipe lasts a really long time because you don't have to keep applying it and because it sinks in and repairs the damage while it moisturizes and protects. No exaggeration!

If you already checked out the ingredients, you also may have guessed that Mike wrote this recipe. Our skin-care notebook is full of side notes on some of my creative accidents that read, for a rinse-out hair conditioner: "hair-brained…way too greasy", or for an oatmeal face scrub, "explosive and shitty!" The face scrub blew its top one day and covered the bathroom in, you guessed it, a baby poop-like substance. We're not making that one anymore!

Our recipe yields enough for 50 tubes. You may ask yourself, what you're going to do with 50 tubes of lip balm. Once your friends find out how good it is, you'll be wondering what happened to all of that lip balm you made.

Lip Armor

66 grams beeswax
44 grams coconut oil
12 grams virgin organic Shea butter
8 grams menthol
20 drops lemongrass
1 large dropper-full camphor

If you don't think you can get some of these ingredients but want to still try your own calming lip balm, try this recipe.

Lip Calm

3 oz. beeswax
2 tablespoons coconut oil
1 ¼ tablespoons almond oil
3 tablespoons Shea butter
30 drops peppermint essential oil

Repurpose any tiny jars or tubes you may have saved if you don't want to invest in new cosmetic tubes and the tube tray you'll need to fill them.

* Please note that these recipes are offered for your personal use on a small-scale. All product names are proprietary to the author.

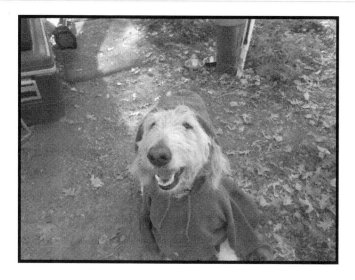

19. PLAY
February 8, 2014

It is 10:42 on a Saturday morning and I am still in bed. The outside temperature is minus two and it is sixty-two inside. Mike and I have been up since 6:30 but are busy constructing a 1000 piece puzzle that is almost an exact replica of the log cabin we are building for ourselves. Like our home, the puzzle cabin is nestled in a few feet of snow, there's a fire going and the warm colors of sunlight bathe the snow in shades of gold and pink. Tiny diamond lights sparkle in the sunlight and Mike comments that we live in a puzzle.

The obvious metaphor makes me chuckle as we have joked about how building our log cabin home has been almost as difficult as assembling this puzzle. I experience a moment of panic, "It's already 11:00 and we haven't even started the projects we intended to get to this weekend!" With sunset at 4:45, we didn't have too many hours left for our to-do list.

In his inimitable way, Mike encouraged me to relax and enjoy the beauty of the moment. *Quite true*, I thought, *there is always time to work. What we really need to work on is more time to play.*

Play is what got us here. When we decided to experience the ultimate in play-dates together, Mike and I fell in love with Northern Maine. Ten days of paddling and camping, getting dirty then bathing in a river, and ending the day with a full appetite go a long way to making you feel like a kid again. Aside from a few adult moments when we weren't completely sure about the map and its directions, we spent all ten days in playful abandon.

Getting there required some planning, true. Play is serious business. We worked pretty hard to make sure we had enough money for the right equipment. But the only way to know what equipment we would need was to play it all out. We took some practice camping trips with our kayaks before we set out on our adventure, 150 miles from the nearest first aid station, much less major hospital. Play doesn't mean you lose your mind and go whole hog into a life-threatening situation with adolescent haste. It means that you have fun in everything you do and your end game is always a little adventurous.

We are able to be playful with life because we have taken care of all the serious stuff already. But even doing that must be fun or we won't do it. Mike likes to say that his world is a sandbox and everyone in it is here for his amusement. It sounds self-serving but everyone who meets him will agree that he not only cares about the people he knows (even casual acquaintances) but without fail will brighten their day with a reason to laugh. Mike knows no strangers.

While travelling in Milan with my family, we were approached by a man wearing a large sign that read "Free Hugs". Being tourists in a crowded mall, everyone in our group avoided any eye contact with this crazy fool who most likely was a pickpocket. Not my husband. He ran straight towards the man, a kindred spirit, and gave him the biggest hug he probably has ever received. The man laughed uncontrollably.

"If he puts his hand in my pocket, all the better!" he said when he returned to us. We all laughed too and the atmosphere of the mall lifted.

Traveling with a light heart and making people laugh,

even people who don't speak your language, is a great way to live. People are attracted to Mike's playful attitude. As a result, in our new home, we have made some very good friends. Of course, I have to take some credit, as we make a good team. Small towns, I have found, are full of friendly people but not always friends. That has not been the case for us. Mike's humor and genuine love of people and our constant prayer to be of service communicates itself to people's hearts and they respond in sincerity. It is lovely and has been helpful.

What I have learned about play is how important it is to our work. Mike and I have completed three 1,000-piece puzzles so far this winter. I would estimate that all together we have spent at least seventy-five hours in bed constructing puzzles. So far we have handled 2,999 pieces. (We still haven't found that darned missing piece.) If that seems like a lot of wasted time, consider this: we have become much more efficient in our work together and get a lot more done as a result.

Playing together has made us realize that we approach problem-solving in two very distinct ways but have noticed that the two ways are complementary. While Mike concentrates fully on an area of the puzzle, I have a tendency to scan all of the areas, seemingly with no purpose in mind. He develops a system of collecting all possible pieces and trying each one, eliminating the pieces that have lines going in the opposite direction, for instance. I scan and settle on a few key missing pieces. I call them transition pieces. You know them. They are the ones that connect two different colors or parts of the puzzle. I scan for a few of these and then search the entire pile for possible fits. It takes some time but is satisfying to my partner as my contribution makes the picture clearer and makes it easier for him to fill in larger sections.

Inevitably Mike will exclaim, "How do you do that?" and I just smile. I'm not sure exactly how I do it but it works.

While working together, Mike will focus in on our project and get the detail work done. I will scan the entire project and note what tools and materials we probably will need. I find them, (digging them out of the snow sometimes), will make sure we have gasoline for the generator, will clear any trip hazards, and will leave enough time to clean up and prepare dinner at the end of the day. I am not, however, good at any of the detail work. I leave that up to Mike and his methodical system-making. He is amazingly efficient.

Understanding each other's work methods makes working together much more fun. Many people have said that building a house together would be the worst thing for our relationship. We say it has been the best thing. We have worked *with* each other, not *against* each other. Working together has congealed our mutual respect and admiration for one another in our hearts and minds.

We have worked hard to create this picturesque log cabin scene we live in, complete with a wood-burning stove and golden lights on the snow. This is true. But play is what we do best. It's our focus, our dream, and how we get it all done.

KOOL-AID TIE- DYE

Playing around with Kool-Aid can make life electric. I'm not suggesting that you drink it though. I think it is much better to use it as a dye for yarn or clothing. Cotton doesn't take the dye the same way other natural fibers like wool, linen, and silk do. But, you can make some beautiful, crazy, fun things with a couple of dollars' worth of Kool-Aid packets. At an average cost of twenty cents each, you can take an old wool sweater and turn it into something new and upbeat that smells good too. If you try it on some old silk scarves or the bottom half of an old silk prom dress, you can make a playful gypsy-style skirt from a few dollars spent at your local "Sally's Boutique" (Salvation Army). The key is to read those tiny labels and to be able to distinguish between silk and polyester or rayon (not always easy, granted).

Use double the amount for vibrant colors, and soak the fiber or fabric in warm water and a couple of tablespoons of vinegar before soaking it in the Kool-Aid.

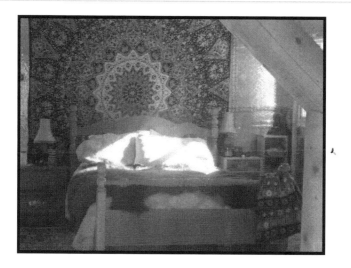

20. REST
February 22, 2014

My father likes to say that a woman's best cosmetic is sleep. There is no doubt in my mind that he is right. It is best not to work too hard on being beautiful; it's best just to rest in the knowledge that you are. True beauty runs deeply through the veins of each of us. Anyone, that is, who can find peace and rest in a world of turmoil. This, I have found, is a lot easier said than done.

What Mike and I have discovered out here on the edge with limited electronic gadgetry (including lights at times) is that we sleep soundly at night and inevitably get a lot of rest. When our bodies are not stimulated by lights, TV, internet, and other electronically dependent activity, we are more prone to listen to what our bodies need and more willing to give in to it.

When winter nights close in at around 4:00, it takes the hounds of hell to try and keep us up past 6:30. We don't even try. In fact, most nights, we're not even sure what time we let go and allow Morpheus to take over. It doesn't matter. We awaken the same way. When the sun rises in the morning, we are ready to go. Our bodies regulate that simple function of our lives. Sleep is the body's territory, we've discovered. It is best to just let it dictate what it needs.

Too many times in our previous lifestyle, we have had to force our bodies to get up and perform prematurely. An alarm clock is such an egregious invention. Just think of it for a moment. It's an alarm. Enough said. Even if you couch it in soft, relaxing music, it is *still* an alarm.

So, how do you maintain a functioning work life without that 5:00 a.m. regimental blast? Can you? Yes, we have found. Better than ever. The brain works better when you give it the chance to listen to its partner, the body.

One of the ways that I have practiced synchronizing my mind with my body is to incorporate the teachings of yoga in my life. Before moving from Rhode Island, when I still had a little income to spend on myself, I trained to be a yoga instructor. I did it mostly because I wanted to deepen my own practice. Since I was moving to a sparsely populated area, I figured I might have to be my own teacher. I was right.

What I didn't expect is that there were several people in my local town who were patiently waiting for a yoga instructor to show up. That's how I ended up with my Monday night classes at the Town Hall. For me it is literally an answer to my prayers. I truly feel that I am of service to my community by leading a yoga class for some of its key members. So, my work life requires no alarm clock anymore. I obviously don't bring home a large paycheck with my new occupation, but the funny thing is, it's enough.

Yoga, as many of you may already know, unifies mind, body and spirit. It is the ultimate power workout because of that alignment. After a good yoga practice, you can't help but feel the *joie de 'vivre* that gives you an overall sense of peace and rest.

When we are in alignment, obstacles become blessings, stillness is not stagnation, and movement becomes prayer. Perhaps it is merely the kind of rest that a person must be ready to experience. Perhaps the practice of yoga is what has made us ready. But I know I can rest in the knowledge that I am a happier person because of my yoga practice. And that is beautiful.

Zzzz… ESSENTIAL OIL MIX

My youngest daughter and I came up with this idea one day as we were mixing essential oils in our kitchen. The beauty is in the simplicity of each component but it works wonderfully to calm the nerves and relax the muscles so that the body can rest. Among many of its properties, lavender is a powerful relaxant, bergamot is a tonic for nerves (wonderful for anxiety and depression), and sage helps the mind stay focused.

Using a small dark glass bottle, place a base of almond, or other fine oil of your choosing, leaving room for the added essential oils. Add a ratio of 2 lavender, 1 bergamot, 1 sage. (Bergamot is also called Bee Balm. If you can't find bergamot, use another citrus oil that isn't too sweet – grapefruit might work). That would mean if you added 12 drops of the lavender, add six drops of the other oils.

Rub a few drops on your forehead, base of neck, and massage into wrists before bed. Surround yourself with a bubble of light and count your blessings instead of sheep.

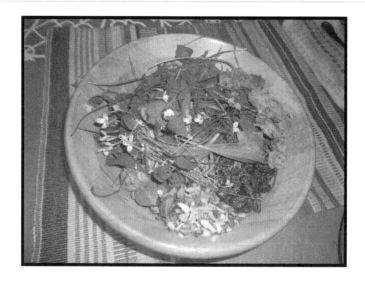

21. TRADE
March 3, 2014

For a handful of years now, Mike and I have been a part of the Maine Primitive Gathering that is held in Wells, Maine. Like most gatherings of kindred spirits, it's an exciting weekend of learning and sharing for us. It was at one of these gatherings that we met Arthur Haines, a remarkable educator and expert forager. Mike and I had been taking baby steps to add more foraged foods to our diet. We had never considered why foraging is such a good idea until we heard Arthur speak at the gathering.

That was also the year that I cleaned up at the trade blanket. To explain, the trade blanket is a place where we all bring something to trade which we place in front of us if we desire the item that is in the middle of the blanket. The person who owns the item in the middle can choose anything from around the circle, ask for more, or can decline any offers. Any trade that is accepted is sealed with a look in the eyes, a handshake, and the words, "Good trade!" It's a great deal of fun and a nice way to exchange goods and knowledge. That year, my autumn olive jam was a big hit and I took back a lot of useful bounty for the small price of twelve little jars. The funny thing is that when I loaded them into our car before the gathering I thought, "No one is going to want these; no one knows what autumn olives are. But, I'm going to bring them anyway because I have a lot of them and I can't give them away!"

Years back, we learned about autumn olive from one of Mike's golfing buddies from Jamestown, Rhode Island. Since that October, we have added many new species to our foraging journeys, breaking the barriers between human consumption and nature's gifts.

Keeping a garden, I have learned, is a lot like being on a seesaw with Mother Nature. She weighs a lot more so we have to expend a lot of energy to keep it going. Most days, we end up flying off if we aren't careful. Between clearing the land, preparing the soil, planting a lot of seeds, nursing the seedlings, weeding out the unwanted growth, trimming the sucker leaves, covering and uncovering raised beds against cold, wind, and rain, and battling the pests, man engages in a constant struggle with nature. Nature is a heavy-weight contender, for sure. Speaking of heavy, do you have any idea how much a groundhog can eat? It always seems to me that while people have been doing it for years, conventional farming is simply inefficient.

Lately I have been hearing more and more about permaculture. It makes perfect sense that if we work in a cooperative relationship with nature, we might have better chances. I'd rather have the heavy-weight on my team than against me. Of course, like all ideas, the new must be tempered with the old and established for optimum results. The only thing is, foraging is a much older form of gaining our sustenance than farming. So which is the old and which is the new?

The way Mike and I look at it, we are willing to learn as much as we possibly can about what is edible in our natural landscape before we tear it all apart to plant new things. We plant and tend to some raised beds but have a healthy respect for what is already planted to tell us its story. Foraging is exciting since it is a discovery of the gifts from our Mother. Her gifts need not be planted, tended, or protected from insects. We need only be willing to learn and allow.

We can move into a more active relationship with Mother Nature like some of our friends do, and spread the plantings. Last year they planted Jerusalem artichoke in as many spots as possible, giving away buckets of the roots to all of their friends. This approach appeals to me since it is a working relationship with nature.

In terms of soil, if it already grows in an acidic soil, then no doctoring needs to be done. We can relegate our tinkering to the narrow strips of raised beds we form and leave the rest alone. In terms of sun, we prefer to work around the spots of shade, recognizing that a little shade is good but too much won't help our cultivated plots. As for sufficient water, small areas are easier to manage than larger swaths. Nature's permanent culture will remain so in our landscape. It needs no fuss.

In terms of nutrition, well, there's no label on a milkweed or a stinging nettle. There's only history to tell us that one is good for getting in some protein and the other for iron. If there were a labelling system for our wild foraged food, it might read: "Only small amounts needed for complete benefit. This food is 100% organic; no pesticides; no fertilizers; no animals were displaced or harmed to produce it; no fossil fuels were expended to gather and process it (unless we drove to its location); all nutrients are naturally derived and combined for maximum absorption; and my personal favorite: no GMO's.

Of course, if you listen to Arthur Haines, who is possibly the leading authority on the subject, you will understand how important it is that we pause and listen to nature and stop trying to tell her how it's done. Our recklessness is a direct result of hubris. So many of our diseases (I think of it as dis- ease) is due to the fact that we are walking around completely malnourished. We eat more because we aren't getting the nutrients our bodies crave. Our bodies are telling us that all of the manipulations we are doing to produce bigger, better, more pest-resistant foods are actually creating foods that simply are not feeding us. We might feel full but our bodies go unsatisfied.

So, why not forage? Why not allow the permaculture to flourish? It is a slower process, no doubt. There aren't too many spots on the planet that haven't been touched by man in some way at some point in history. But, why not allow small chunks of land go fallow? Why not let weeds grow in?

What are weeds? What we define as weeds might just be the most valuable plants you can allow to grow. If left to express herself, Mother Nature is resplendent with wisdom. In the absence of lawn seed, fertilizers, and pesticides, what will grow in your front yard: dandelion: a great salad green, tea to cleanse the liver, coffee substitute for vigor rather than nerves; stinging nettle (already mentioned for iron and blood restorative), wood sorrel good for salads; red clover flowers for a nice Vitamin C pick-me-up tea, plantain (the weed, not the fruit), a delicious fresh and cooked green and a miraculous salve when infused in olive oil. The list goes on and on. In fact, once you start to learn what grows wild, you realize how foolish the whole process of weeding out weeds truly is.

Of course, once we begin to shift our tastes and begin putting more foraged foods on our plates, it might have an adverse effect on the big chemical and food monopolies (no need to mention them, you know which ones I mean). We would never want to do that, I'm sure.

Being a natural born dreamer, my mind drifts to a new victory garden. It is one that is in harmony with nature, one that needs no tending. The only thing it needs is neighbors and housing associations to recognize that the wild and weedy patch of growth you are allowing to grow in your yard IS your garden: your right to eat what you want and allow things to grow. Perhaps if enough of us tried it, it would become the "new, trendy" thing to do and we might have common areas in our housing plats that are allowed to go wild. The gravelly, turned-up soil creates a perfect environment for these beneficial plants. Think about the simplicity of it.

I am convinced that small is the way things happen best. Small steps are careful, thoughtful steps. Small steps lead us to more steps. It just happens that way. Tasting the sunshine in a dandelion flower is really cool. Batter fry it in butter and olive oil and take a walk on the wild side.

While gardening is good exercise, foraging is better still. When we forage, we walk and hike, we bend and crawl, and breathe fresh oxygen. It is better for our spirits too since we are grateful to Mother Nature, not cursing her for blights and pests. Overall, I see it as a beautiful complement to the benefits of gardening.

Every year we gather with our Maine Primitive friends in Wells, we are met with a heated anticipation of our autumn olive jam. We have branched out and made a fruit leather which is coveted by young and old and we love to put the berries in our morning smoothies too since I have observed that they are also are a noticeable cleanser for the digestive tract. I don't need a scientific study or a label to know that this food is good for me.

While avid gardeners are cursing the autumn olive for crowding out their carefully-placed cultivations, Mike and I (and a growing number of others) are blessing Mother Nature for providing such an abundant, healthy, and resilient food source for the simple price of learning her ways. Another reason classical gardeners may try to obliterate this wondrous weed is that critters love it too. Keeping the critters fed is just another motivation for broadcasting its seeds all around the inhospitable periphery of our gravelly road bed. It should be happy up here where no one will bother it.

As for the reasons we are adding more and more foraged foods to our dinner plates, well, it is all part of the realization that as we reconnect more and more to the Natural Grid on a physical level, we are also connecting on an emotional and spiritual level. Mother Nature is calling us to reconnect to her gifts and realize that we are best served to act in a spirit of cooperation with her rather than competition. We all know which party will eventually win.

RUNNING A TRADE BLANKET

I first learned about a trade blanket from a teacher at the Maine Primitives School Gathering in Wells, Maine. I wish I could remember who the teacher was so that I could extend the credit but like all useful ideas, it's more important that we share than that we own. I can just tell you that the trade blanket brings people together in an unusually deep way and satisfies the human desire for something new and the need for clearing out. Some people think about the trade blanket all year.

The moderator (preferably an elder who desires nothing new) lays out a blanket. All participants circle the blanket with something/s they would like to trade away. Each person takes a turn placing an item or items in the middle of the blanket and if participants in the circle want to trade an item for what is offered, they place their item on the blanket. The person who is "up" decides if he/she wants any of the trades offered.

If the trade is agreeable, both parties shake hands, look each other in the eye, and say, "Good trade." The trade is sealed. I have seen weighty silver necklaces from Greece being traded for a few jars of foraged homemade jam. I have seen a bundle of dried sticks and a homemade basket be traded for a good camp stove. Both parties leave astonishingly happy about their trades and good friendships are forged over the trade blanket. Kind gestures and loving hearts abound as young and old trade more than items; they trade knowledge. Those dried sticks teach the new owner what willow looks and feels like and the basket is a model of what the sticks can become. If the new owner is interested, the old owner will tell him how it's done. It is truly exciting and well-worth the price of an old stove.

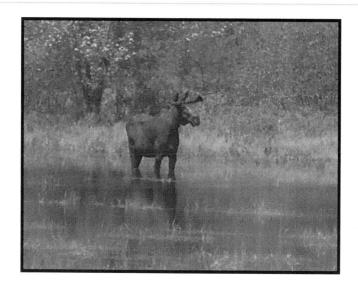

22. MOOSEGRASS
March 4, 2014

The river is still frozen and I feel pretty certain it will remain so through most of the month of March, right up into April. We have experienced a pretty cold winter and my instincts tell me that the weather will be slow to change this year. I have learned to listen closely to my inner guidance. It is almost always more accurate than the weatherman. Ever since that memorable afternoon on Lake Chamberlain on the Allagash Waterway, Mike has learned to listen to my little expressions about the weather too.

"There's some strange winds coming our way. I think we ought to head to shore," I shouted to Mike across the distance between our two kayaks. I usually deferred to Mike's knowledge on such matters since he spent many days of his life on open waters as a New England fisherman.

Examining the cloud formations, he said, "Nah, storms never come in from the north. These clouds are circling past us. We won't get hit." After a discerning pause, he said, "But if the temperature drops suddenly we need to paddle as fast as we can to the shore." He indicated exactly where with his paddle.

Within three minutes the temperature dropped dramatically and we both knew we had to paddle hard and fast if we were going to make it to the rocky beach in time. The surface of the lake went from placid mirror to four foot waves within minutes. It took every ounce of energy and strength for us to reach shore, pull out the four foot tarp we had stashed in Mike's hold, and batten it down with heavy rocks around our huddled bodies as a quick lean-to. The wind was unseasonably cold and we were wet. Our lean-to protected us from the cold driving rain for a good forty-five minutes and then the storm cleared as quickly as it came in.

What we learned later that day as we headed for our scheduled stop on the Thoreau Island campsite was that we had a near-miss with a tornado. When we arrived at the campsite, we found a five-foot wide oak completely uprooted and covering the spot where we would have placed our tent. We also discovered that the Boy Scout troop that had been paddling ahead of us had a tough time comprised of capsized canoes and "man-over-boards" because of the sudden and severe weather.

To this day, Mike listens when I say something off-handed about the weather because I am usually right. I don't go by any intellectual knowledge, I just go by the way I feel, and have a much better record than the weather reports.

Paddling the Allagash Waterway taught us to stop and listen and to feel to find our way. We had a hand-drawn photocopy of a map of our trail and a good laminated colored map of the entire region but there were many times when we had to make some choices about which way to go. Choosing the wrong way could mean an hour or two delay in setting up camp which sometimes meant having to tack on an extra couple of hours on the water since the campsite we planned to use was already taken. There are no reservations on the Allagash Waterway, just good timing. And the campsites have capacity-limits to reduce wear and tear on the land.

As most waterway travelers know, you have to make split-second decisions all day long. Life on a river is a careful balance between river and rocks and we soon discovered that if you focus on the rocks, you're sure as heck going to hit them. What we learned from the river is that life is a lot better if you focus on the water, not the rocks. When you do, the river will take you right around the rocks. When you don't, you head straight into them and there's nothing the river can do but push you harder in that direction. As in life, too many collisions with rocks can be painful.

Skiers will relate. Just go with the flow. It's safer and much more pleasant. Sounds pretty easy but there's some little tickling part of human nature that plays a siren's song with our emotions and before we know it, we're all tangled up and have hit hard.

Sometimes the hard hits happen in lots of little bits. Mike and I discovered that it can be painful when you choose the wrong side of a river to paddle. Before you know it, you've hit a bony, scrabbly part that won't support even the three-inch draw of your kayak and you have to get out and portage over the rocks, sometimes for more than an hour, before you can get back to the flow again. This process is hard on your feet. Even if you have good water shoes, the gravelly river bottom finds its way into your shoes and jabs at all the tender spots. It's definitely something to avoid if possible.

What we learned from the dry patches of our river trail is that looking below the surface of the water can tell you where to go. What you will see is the light green moose grass that resembles a mermaid's hair and it will flow in the direction of the river. Like strands of hair, it will be straightest in the direction of the strongest flow. It's a simple observation that saved us many a narrow bottleneck that would have ended in pain and wasted energy.

Following the moose grass has become our mantra for life. When scanning the many ways to make an income or ways to spend personal energy, we refer back to the idea. Listen and observe the obvious. Stop and take the time to listen to how you feel. Pay attention to the indicators. Nature has many languages and we all speak at least one of those. Perhaps it is a feeling in the gut, a chill in the bones, a whisper, a crow's call, or a formation in the clouds. Nature, like the river, will show us the right way. If we follow the flow and avoid the siren's song of doubt and skepticism, we will probably avoid wasted energy and frustration.

We could also avoid weathering a tornado on open water or pitching a tent up on the spot where a ten-ton tree is going to fall. Many times, following the moose grass, listening to the wind, looking up, and waiting to see what Nature's creatures have to say to me has proven a much better source of information than the standard weather report. I'll still keep my wind-up weather radio, but for a complete picture, I stop and listen to nature's language. It's got a better record with me.

PACKING FOR THE ALLAGASH

If you're going to take the entire trip, it could take you about ten days. That includes camping on some of the lower lakes and then paddling through the upper lakes until you reach the river and taking the river all the way north to the town of Allagash.

You have to figure that you'll want to keep your load light because even if you're in a canoe, you will have to portage sometimes. If you go with guides, they might be willing to take your beer but, they'll probably charge you more because it takes a lot of energy and manpower to portage cases of beer. That goes for other things too. Remember, whatever you bring in you have to either eat or take out. You can burn most packaging but probably don't want to burn plastic and certainly don't want to be the first person to leave your litter there.

So, that's why Mike and I decided to learn how to dehydrate our food. Being the frugal sort, we couldn't see spending large bills on dehydrated food that was processed in a factory. We wanted choices and wanted to fuel our bodies since they are the engines for our boats.

We learned right away that packaged foods that contain too much salt are not what you need at the end of a day paddling. Many of the commercial meals you buy in the outdoor shops are loaded with salt. Having said that, your body will need some salt but it needs it in little amounts throughout the day rather than all at once in a meal. Having a trail mix with raisins, salted peanuts, and some m&m's thrown into whatever other nuts and dried fruit you have is helpful for your salt/potassium/protein/blood sugar balancing act. The lack of these can bring on serious fatigue (or in the case of my husband, some grumpiness) and that can lead to dangerous trail errors.

The best way to pack your food is to make double portions of your dinners for two weeks and then dehydrate your leftovers. The first two days you eat your fresh foods, the next two days, you eat your frozen meals, then for the remainder of your trip, you get to enjoy all of your dehydrated efforts.

Our favorite dehydrated meal is lasagna, made exactly the way you would with cheese, meat, and all. We found that it is best to soak the meal in water for a good 45 minutes and then heat it in your Jet boil. If your sauce is a little watery, you can add some tomato bark. We'll get to that in a minute. We have read that some people like to cook the pasta on site and then add it to the lasagna mixture. We're going to try that next time out. We'll let you know how it comes out.

And now for the culinary aspirin: it makes everything better. You cook your pasta, retain the water, add your tomato bark (made in advance by dehydrating tomato sauce like you would make fruit leather), stir, and *voila!* Pasta with your own homemade sauce. Take that Chef Boy-r-d! Good food on the trail is very important.

Making sure you pack treats, good, hearty ones like apple cobblers that you can warm up at the end of the day is also important. Cookies, once again, can serve as valuable currency with fellow travelers. Right around day six, I was willing to let our friends in the boy scout troop play around in my precious kayak for the trade of one good oatmeal cookie. Next time, I'm holding the gold!

What we do spend some money on is our equipment. Getting light becomes an obsession. Our down sleeping bags are so small, they could fit in a coffee can. Our tent weighs less than two pounds. We purchased self-inflating sleeping pads that roll up. We also spent money on heavy-duty dry bags. You also want to bring along a fire rod and know how to use it. There's plenty of firewood right around the campsites so a collapsible bow saw comes in handy. Save your money on fire-starters by soaking cotton balls in melted Vaseline. They make fire starting very easy and they don't mind getting wet.

We brought along, Gilpatrick's *Guide to the Allagash* so we would not miss any of the sights. (Hint: there's a full-sized train just sitting out there in the middle of the wilderness.) His guide also offers tips about where to camp and how to make sure you secure your site. All campsites are first-come-first-served and can't accommodate more than two small groups. It's very important to schedule your paddles so you leave enough time and energy to find another campsite if the one you planned on using is full. It happens.

My gypsy upbringing has taught me to always pack a lot of bandanas. They come in handy in a lot of ways, including cooling off your head when you start to get dehydrated and you don't have time to stop and filter water. Oh yeah, we used the Katahdin Water filter with good results since it provides enough water for drinking and cooking.

A 10x10 tarp for your occasional tornado is always handy. Just in case. Keep your clothing light-weight and easy to dry but make sure you have layers because it can get cold out there at night. Avoid cotton clothing. You'll lose a lot of body heat waiting for it to dry. A **thin** wool layer is worth its weight in gold.

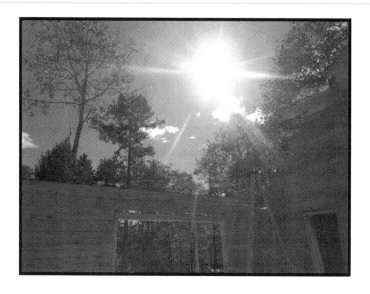

23. NATURAL GRID
March 6, 2014

Mike and I are not out here trying to make a point. We had just reached a point. We had reached a point where we needed to simplify and are doing it. When we bought our land up here, we weren't thinking that it was going to be a permanent residence. We thought we would camp on it and eventually build a small house for vacations. We knew it would have to be off-grid since running electricity this far off-road would cost us close to $20,000. We thought it might have a well but knew that the river water would be sufficient if we didn't.

The first few years of camping on our property we used a ceramic dome filter and a five gallon pail to set up an excellent water filtering system. We never lacked potable water. It rains a lot up here. We also always camped in warmer weather, except for the time we camped in February in our teardrop trailer and the snow was about three feet deep. The camper has no heat but it blocked the wind and snow enough so that our super warm sleeping bags and a sizeable buffalo robe thrown over us, kept us toasty warm. We look back to that time as one of the best we have shared here.

Lately I have been thinking that when my days are warm and easy and I have plenty of money and resources to buy and do as I wish, my memories are not quite as crisp. So too with my toughest days. I remember them, but the corners around the snapshots are hazy. There might appear an object or a face, a feeling, but the complete picture is lost. My best memories are of days that are somewhere in between. Days when I was not particularly dependent on anything material, might have been just a little hungry, and had found meaning in the quiet of solitude or in the company of friends.

The one thing that all of these crystalline images have in common is that I am relaxed enough to allow the taproot of my energy field to dig deep into the earth and connect with nature, like a large umbilical cord. I felt at one with all things on the planet, whether they be rock, river, tree, insect, or mammal. To use a term I first encountered in one of Alberto Villoldo's books, I felt myself reconnected to the Natural Grid.

Though Mike is a much more pragmatic person, he responds the same way I do to nature. We share the need to reconnect as much as possible. When people ask, we find ourselves saying that we just love nature and are driven by the need to be as close as possible to her and her glory. We would rather be more connected to the Natural Grid than to the Industrial Grid.

This doesn't mean that we don't do technology. In fact, we both have cell phones and internet access. We both go into town for work and commodities like Laundromat, library, and grocery store but we are not so connected that we are lost or bored without these things. We do not live in fear of being snowed in for days, or even weeks if it happens, but we bought a plow truck to get us out so we don't have to.

We don't live in fear of the animals on our property. At night we have heard coyote, wolf, and something really big and powerful that jumped out from behind the wood pile that Mike never saw, but felt, as he brought in a load of wood one night. Well, I have to say that he ran back into the house as fast as he could when it happened. I guess that does count as a natural-born fear of something. The next day we saw the snow tracks where it had attacked a flock of turkeys, that's what Mike heard. The predator prints looked like they could be lynx. The turkey prints were all scattered and afraid. This week we found some four-inch-wide feline prints that we were able to cast in plaster. They are impressive, no doubt. Most of our resident experts say Mountain Lion. There are web-cam pictures to support their claims. It's pretty darned big and could take down our dog in a heartbeat. That's why I carry my gun when I am out and about. There's no fooling around with this rule.

All I need is for my dog to get into a scuff with one of these big guys or our resident bear and we'll have a mess on our hands. My plan with the gun is to shoot over their heads to scare the large animal off. If it doesn't, well, that's why it's important to target shoot.

EDIBLE FLOWERS

Flowers are Mother Nature's public relations department. They are the movers and shakers that demand our attention. Most of us think that plants stay put. If you have ever tried to track mullein, you are well-aware that plants do move! You'll swear there was an entire row in a spot last year and they will have disappeared, only to reappear somewhere else. That's why weed-walkers know how to spot the difference between a first year plant and a second year plant.

Make sure before you forage for any wild plants that you have checked not only with books, online resources, but also with a seasoned weed-walker. The plants I am listing here are common in most back yards and open spaces and are easily identified.

I'll start with the dandiest of them all, the dandelion. For an absolute flavor treat, try batter frying these yellow pom-poms in a little olive oil and butter. Roll them in seasoned flour (I like Italian herbs, salt, and pepper). Fry them in a small amount of butter and olive oil.

You'll never think of early spring the same way again. You'll treat those "weeds" like the princess flowers they truly are and wouldn't consider ever feeding them weed-killer again. The flowers must be cooked right after you pick them. Dandies wait for no one! The young leaves are beneficial as a salad green. The roots may be used as a coffee substitute and the entire plant is a wonderful cleaning product for our body's housekeeping department: the kidneys and liver.

Violets are also a little treat. I have used them for my cordials but enjoy them most in my spring salad. The color boost cannot be overlooked since eating is a multi-sensory experience and color is an important aspect of our nourishment. We find wild violas on our property. They are purple-blue and low-lying. Looking for them encourages a hike outside when I need it most.

Along with chive, which produces a nice little garlic-flavored light purple flower, I plant nasturtium seeds in my garden and planters. The flowers are blaze orange and promise a zesty flavor surprise. The tender, light green leaves are round and add a peppery bounce to your salad bowl also. They do have a tendency to volunteer in your garden the following years so they might be considered perennials, I'm not sure. I think it depends on the climate. The chives **are** perennial though.

Another flower I cherish for eating is the squash flower. Ever since my friend Al told me that his Italian grandmother used to batter fry them for him when he was a kid, ("Like candy!" he said), I have always planted a lot of zucchini in my garden, mostly for the flowers. Make sure you pick the male flowers. They are the ones with a long stalk. The female flowers turn into the fruit so their stalks will have a fuller, rounder shape.

Though the seeds of plantain flower stalks are edible, the leaves are most commonly what we use from the plant. The useful benefits of plantain are so numerous that it requires its own chapter. (See Book II for that or preempt my strategy and look it up. You'll be amazed.) As a salad green, plantain is slightly sweet and voluminous. This comes in handy since most foraged salad greens have a tendency to be flat and slightly bitter. Plantain leaves give your salad a noticeable lift.

While we are at it, milkweed flowers are wonderful too. I like to harvest the green flower buds. They are similar to broccoli in some ways. If you batter fry them like you do with the dandelions, they are quite tasty. Some people use them in a stir-fry. Cook them any way you would a green vegetable and you won't be disappointed.

The flowers are also edible when they blossom. They smell much like lilacs (which are edible too, by the way!). Flowers may be eaten raw but, since some people have a bit of sensitivity to the latex in the milkweed plant, it might be best to cook them. It won't kill you to try it either way.

If nothing else, probably the number one reason to eat flowers is that it makes for a good motive to go for a hike.

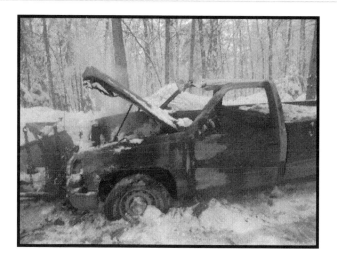

24 LIFE AS AN ADVENTURE
March 10, 2014

Today I celebrated the advent of spring by going for a hike with Hermes. The only thing is, I had to strap on snowshoes before heading out, since the snow is still four to five feet deep in the woods and where we didn't plow. Speaking of plowing, we were forced to stop plowing last month after a storm dropped twenty-two inches on our already deep build-up. Struggling to keep up, Mike had been plowing all morning and was about half-way through getting our long driveway under control, when our plow truck burst into flames and took hours to put out.

Since we are a good distance off the main road in a pretty rural part of Maine, it took the fire department almost an hour to arrive and they couldn't get their fire truck onto our road so they came to watch us finish up by shoveling snow into the truck's engine. The plow truck burnt to the ground. The firemen did help us figure out what had happened, though. They explained that the hydraulic fluid of the plow has a low flash point so when it leaks onto the engine block, it almost always catches fire. The old rusty truck we bought for the plow had been losing parts all winter long and it had finally called it quits. By all accounts, it was a pretty tough winter for everyone.

As a result, we have been walking more than half a mile to get to our cars which are parked near the main road. Mornings aren't so bad but nights have been tough since we have been trekking on icy, patchy, sometimes puddly terrain and we can't always see where we are stepping. Add to that scenario whatever work bag, bundle of tools, lunch, gas can, propane tank, laundry, or other necessities and you get the picture. Suffice it to say, winter really kicked our butts this year. Our reserves are worn thin in every area of our lives but we are the happiest we have ever been.

Recently, I have begun working as a substitute teacher in a local high school. This morning I was not called in to work so I walked with Mike to his work van at the end of the road. The walk gave us some peaceful time together. We commented that many people grind through fifty weeks of routine in order to have two weeks to do exactly what we were doing at that moment: taking a walk through the woods with a dog who is free to roam at will. There are many who pay heavily for the chance to feel free and at peace with nature and they usually have to share it with a lot of other people all doing it at the same time.

Mike was heading in to our friend's auto shop to work on our jeep, something we would need for mud season, less than two weeks away. We rescued our daughter's jeep. The 1997 Wrangler was the car she worked hard to buy while in high school. When it stopped running, her plan was to sell it for junk. To be fair, it had too many problems for her to be able to fix.

Mike took a look at it and we developed a plan. We couldn't bear to see all of her hard work end up in scraps. As it turned out, most of what it needed was labor-intensive but did not require a lot of new parts. He rebuilt the engine in the living room last month and has just a few things left to do. He is finishing it up in our friend's garage in exchange for helping him get his cars on the road again. This winter has been tough on all vehicles.

It is imperative that we both know how to fix and make the things we need. The plow truck is beyond fixing so we will have to buy a new one. We will have to save for it over the summer. This means picking up a little more work and being efficient so as to get things done swiftly to pick up more work. It means a little more effort and a lot more care when spending money but we will come up with a plan and stick to it. That's how we have managed to do everything else. The plow truck is just another bump in the road, (a bump in the road IS a bump in the road!) a pretty big one, granted, but we have faith in each other and the Universe that what we need will appear when we are ready.

When we talk about the burning of the truck, we speak in terms of gratitude that no one was hurt and that the fire did not reach the house. We remind each other of the lessons it taught us. We learned that we have to be prepared to be our own emergency response team, that we need bigger and better fire extinguishers, and need to rethink our other emergency supplies, including a solid first aid kit. We also are reminded that safety is still number one, even though we aren't cutting trees, up on makeshift scaffolding, or working on an icy roof.

It doesn't matter where you live or who you are, life is full of risks. We just happen to be a little farther from outside help than people who live in larger towns. The trade-off is that we get to hear and see nature all of the time without the interruption of traffic, sirens, voices, and all of the other clutter that accompanies populated places.

Out here, we are the incidentals, not wild animals. This morning I heard all manner of birds talking including the gobble of a flock of turkeys, the caw of blue jays, the chirp of chickadees. Last night an owl visited us, perched outside our bedroom window. I know this happens in the suburbs too but with all of the clutter, we don't always get to notice. Out here, noticing it is the norm, not the occasional. What is occasional is the sound of a jet airplane overhead or the whistle of the train as it passes through our nearby town. Depending on the season, we may hear the hum of snowmobiles and four-wheelers or the buzz of a chain saw and the roar of a truck loaded with trees headed to the mill.

This week, the predominant sound has been the river as it begins its seasonal melt. The colors of the river range from aquamarine-blue to lemon-green on a moving background of whites and browns as the giant shards of ice begin to break away. We are all praying for a slow melt since an ice jam on the river could cause flooding on the roads.

Mike and I have a readiness plan in case there is an ice jam. Out here where we live, we could get stranded for some days during the melt since there are a few low spots on the roads and by the bridges. The roads are already closed to the big logging trucks and are replete with potholes that could swallow a moose.

This winter will go down as a record-breaker and we couldn't be happier that it was our first. Mike and I readily admit that if we had experienced a mild first winter, we might feel a little too confident about our abilities and might accuse locals of exaggerating the impact of winter on their lives. People up here are obsessed with the weather because it rules.

One of our neighbors works in the records department of the hospital two towns over. She misses two weeks a year because of mud season. Because of the heavy snowfall this winter, we are all expecting it will be a tough mud season and probably a good one for the black flies. Nature doesn't fool around but she sometimes will fool you. It could just as easily be the shortest mud season too. There's really no telling. It all depends on how much sun, how much rain, and all of the other stuff that determines overall weather conditions.

I think my neighbor has it right. When the roads get too difficult to travel, stay home and knit a sweater for next winter. When our car (a four wheel drive 2003 Honda CRV) lost its guts on chunks of ice sticking up on our road two weeks ago, we were down to only being able to use Mike's work van. Like I said, winter kicked our butts.

So far, our transition to our new life up here has not been easy but it sure has been an adventure. Fortunately, Mike and I both share a deep-felt need for adventure. We were only willing to trade a controlled lifestyle, with reliable vehicles and consistent income for the period of time it took to raise the kids.

It was a commitment we made to normalcy but we both knew we could only hold up for so long before we died of persistent tedium.

Every life has its parts that fall off. But for us, the cost of holding together all of the creature comforts of turning on a light any time of day or night, ample room to store things that creep into every corner of a house and dressing for success every day of the week cost way too much for us. Mike and I share the need to fly free and meet each day as a separate event with its own agenda while expecting the unforeseen. We need to anticipate life, wondering if this could be the day, or event, that goes down in history as the funniest story ever.

We could never settle into a daily routine of a night of favorite TV shows, a comfortable chair, and a fridge full of packaged, prepared food. We couldn't survive on factory-baked bread or even bread from a high-end bakery. We have to make our own, even if it means going without because we've been too busy on a job that week. We dread eating in restaurants unless it is a really good one and it's a special occasion.

Loaded down with a tank of propane and assorted bags of groceries last week on our half-mile hike home from the van, we noticed some fresh snowshoe tracks heading down our driveway. They were large and whoever it was travelled alone. We figured it was probably made by someone from the camps up river. Our guess was Larry since he often will come up alone to work on his camp.

Sure enough, when we rounded the bend, he came marching up to us with a huge grin on his face. "I have been by four times to try and catch you guys. I saw the truck and thought you might have just given up! I wouldn't blame you. Look at you guys, you made it! You survived this winter. You didn't leave!"

He said that when he saw the fresh dog poop in the driveway, he figured we were still here and he wasn't going to give up until he saw for sure we were okay.

The burnt-up truck is quite a fearful sight. It would make

anyone wonder if we had fled the scene and planned to never come back, that's true. Larry came up to the house and Mike got a fire going in the wood stove. I rustled up some of my homemade hard cider I had been saving in the root cellar and poured out a couple of tiny glasses of my St. John's Wort cordial to toast to our success. We warmed up a little soup and ate some homemade bread. He mentioned how great the house was coming along and we told him the story of how the truck burned.

There's a proximity that occurs between people who like to live life as an adventure. It's a brotherhood that requires no delicacies or posturing. The simple fact that Larry was glad we were still alive, walking hand-in-hand and laughing was enough. Our vehicles were all in various levels of disrepair and we still have to start the generator to take a shower, but we made it. We didn't just survive the toughest winter most Mainers say they have ever seen, we were thriving. We came out shining: smiling, laughing, and grateful for each day that we share together.

That I can wake up each day next to my soul mate and dedicate myself to the dream I have had since I was a child in my grandparents' living room, to write my stories in a simple house in the woods, is a priceless gift. The fact that I can decide to hike with my dog today because the colors of the river are uniquely beautiful and the sun is dancing brightly on the powerful streams of dark water that have broken free from the chunks of ice, makes my life an adventure.

I just couldn't miss it.

A WELL-DESIGNED OUTHOUSE

The funny thing about life is that it is full of poopy situations. I have known people who specialize in poop. I think that's great. One thing about being wild and living life as an adventure is, you have to know what to do with the crap or it could make your adventure a nasty mess and that's no fun.

When it was just the two of us camping on the property, Mike and I had our "spots" and would dig a hole. That's fine for a couple of days but if you camp for more than that and if you bring along your dog, you might need to pack a good pair of rubber gloves and use a lot of soap and water. Not my ideal adventure, I can tell you.

So that's why Mike decided to build an outhouse for the property. He needed to build it in our yard in Rhode Island and transport it on our utility trailer to the property since we didn't have the tools or the power to get it done on site. He built it in parts so that it could be easily disassembled and moved. As usual, he altered the designs he found online and came up with his own system of venting it that is sleek and economical. I like the sleek part because it keeps critters out and is easy to clean. For some reason, spiders love outhouses so the less tubing and hidden corners you create, the easier it is to kick them out.

To make our outhouse inexpensive, lightweight but durable, he used 2X3's and T-111. If you're not sure what that means, get someone else to build it for you. He made a sandwich: using the 2X3's to frame up the exterior walls of T-111 and covered the interior walls with ¼" plywood. The all-important throne was constructed with 3/4'" plywood. The key to an odor-free outhouse is venting. This was accomplished by leaving the bottom one foot section of the back wall of the interior side open (underneath the bench seat) and placing screened vents on the top portion of the exterior back wall. Cap it off with tinted corrugated plastic roofing at a steep angle. This allows for light and our roof held up well under a difficult winter.

When locating your outhouse, dig a deep pit (ours was about four feet deep) and make it so that the back wall faces south. Paint the back wall a darker color to absorb heat. (We camouflaged ours but that did create some problems with folks who couldn't find it!) The sun hitting the back wall will warm the airspace, causing the warmer air to rise, thereby venting the lower collection area beneath the bench. Add TP and say goodbye to one of life's messy situations.

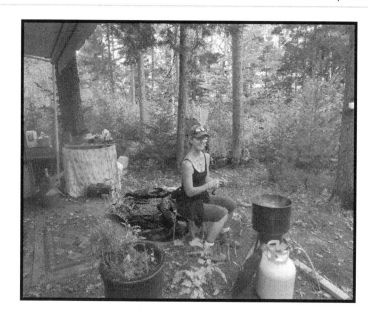

25. THE POWER OF NONE
March 18, 2014

Yesterday, while most adults in Rhode Island were thinking about drinking green beer, Mike and I signed the closing papers on our house. The bottom line was $0.00. It was interesting to note that all parties involved in the transaction made money but us. Eight years ago, we put down $65,000 in cash to buy our house. It was the peak of the housing bubble. We put more than that amount in upgrades during the years we owned the house. Like most, our property values sank about $80,000 in the eight years we owned it. The devaluation was not the result of anything we did wrong. In fact, it happened in spite of everything we did right. It took two years for our house to sell and we finally ended the experience in a short sale.

Yet, we left feeling ecstatically happy. Owing nothing is much better than *owning* much and *owing* for it all. The large house in a bucolic New England town had served its purpose as we raised our daughters and practiced our homesteading skills.

But like a snake shedding its skin, we were finally free of the financial obligations that kept us tangled up in something we no longer could use. We were happy that a bright new family would inhabit its land and love it the way we did.

On the five and a half hour drive back to Maine, my mind scanned all of the many powerful ways that zero manifests itself.

Being a true lover of Emily Dickinson, my mind drifted to her poem, "I am Nobody/ who are you?" I treasure the freedom of being nobody in a world full of shouting somebodies who amount to no more than anyone else when the great director of our lives claims that the play is over. What character did you play? Was it a starring role? Is it worth saving the play's program to immortalize the moments you were on stage? How many lines did you have to memorize? Did you memorize every line and then you never got to play the part because you were just the understudy? How many play programs can you save in life before the stuff you save reaches explosive levels and you don't have any room for any of it anymore? Did you collect so much memorabilia connected to that play that it clogs up the rooms of your house and you can't inhale for all of the dust it creates?

Mike says the pictures on our walls should be its windows, unencumbered by curtains. I have to agree. But what do I do with all of those sentimental things that I have collected over the years? It is time to take a look at it all and consolidate what we need. Organization, I have come to learn, can improve almost anything. But his idea would mean we would have nothing on our walls. An enticing idea, I have to admit.

Nothing, it seems, might be the ultimate solution to too much.

Nothing, zero, neutral, empty, space, void, level ground are all good places. If you start at nothing, the "tabula rasa", you have only one direction for movement. It is the fulcrum for the balancing act of life. To be able to find and maintain neutral position is a gift that experts spend lifetimes trying to accomplish.

Zero is the luminous egg that protects us from both loss and gain. Like a child, able to enter the kingdom of Heaven, we return to the nothingness of experience, to the unknown mystery, able to accept what we don't know, but curious to learn. We reach upward, seeking the warmth of a loving face, the gentle sway of a tree, the light of the sun.

No one can gain anything from you other than what you are willing to give when you are nobody. After all, who wants *nothing* anyway? Only people who have already experienced the chains that *having* puts on them will want nothing from you. And, honestly, at that point, they have already realized that it's not something you can get from anyone else anyway. It's something that must be earned. It takes a lot of effort to earn zero.

Most people never get there in this lifetime. Some people are born with it and spend their time trying to forget it. They expend all of their earthly energy on having something and being someone.

Needing to be someone and have something creates a lot of worry. This can rob people of years of their lives. I know, I have spent lifetimes worrying about everything and losing what I have. Having nothing sinks me deeper into being able to enjoy what I do have: my relationships, my primary reason for being here in the present.

When something costs us no money, we say it is free. So many things are given that label to entice us into all kinds of contractual webs of servitude. We are taught by our elders that there is no such thing as free. This is true. Our freedom has cost us much in the way of effort and determination. For Mike and me, our freedom was not free but we were free all along to seek it. We just weren't aware of it until we awakened from the American Dream as most of us understand it today. Our forefathers created a different American Dream. It was the dream of freedom not of stuff.

Today our neuro-pathways are determined by our closer cultural ancestors to see only one path to freedom and that is through ownership. Mike and I still travel some of those pathways, accepting that we need to be in possession of some important things to survive. We have worked hard to "own" our land and the house on it. Each item we own is something we chose. We didn't allow our stuff to choose us.

Freedom from the American Dream as it has evolved in the last 200 years has prompted us to look at the natural forest of life and see that if we are good at navigation, we do not have to stay on the beaten paths; we can forge new pathways. We can create our own dream, replete with the magic of God and nature and all of the mysteries. We are not sentenced to a life of monotonous cycles of alarm clocks, lunch hours, and rush hour traffic blues to get home to prepare for the next day of it all over again.

Perhaps the greatest realization Mike and I had was that we are free to choose the alarm clock-cycled life if we want to. We don't judge those who *do choose* it. But some point, long ago, after our trip to the Allagash, we both decided that we would choose something else. Seven years ago, we didn't really know what our new choice was going to be. But if there was one thing that our watery pilgrimage taught us, it was that we did have a choice.

I often think about the Zen story of a monk who owned nothing but a loincloth and his wooden begging bowl. On one night of the full moon, a thief, finding the monk in deep meditation, took the opportunity to steal the monk's bowl. Before the thief was able to sneak away, the monk opened his eyes and said, "It is too bad I can't offer you the moon as well, my dear friend. Perhaps you will take my loincloth instead?"

When Mike and I experienced the feeling of belonging to Mother Nature and the Great Spirit on our ten-day paddle seven years ago, we began to feel we don't need much more than that communion. We realize that the script of being exiled from the garden is a choice. We are on the return and the Great Creator seems pleased with our choice. We are not haunted by the feeling of separateness that our modern ancestors have scripted into our neuro-pathways. We belong in the garden and it has what we need.

After signing the house-closing documents yesterday, I was thinking about the Luck of the Irish. I thought about all of the hardships they have had to face and still face every day. Yet, they sing and dance anyway. That is the neuro-pathway their ancestral culture has encrypted into their brains. That and other not so positive stuff, granted. But, they are free to choose which pathways they run. As Americans, we are too.

Once I signed those closing documents, I felt richer than I have ever felt in my life. From the zero I gained that day, I have recovered the vital energy that the sticky web of *owing-ship* was robbing from me. Even the ownership of our simple hand-built camp way up here, too far for electrical hook-up isn't a sticky web.

It carries with it the knowledge that we are able to build again without owing anyone. To our credit, our credit is our ability to rebuild when needed. We can start from zero again any day because we have been there once and we know our way home.

PASTA
(Couch-cushion Gourmet)

It always amazes me how many things a person can make with the same four ingredients: flour, oil, eggs, and milk. Pasta is one of those things. Only it gets away with using three of the four and is a real game-changer when you're down to almost nothing in the cupboard.

Of course, you can buy pasta for next to nothing but it's useful to know how to make it if you run out. Homemade pasta becomes a gourmet meal when tossed in olive oil and dried herbs. The price goes up considerably when you purchase good, fresh pasta in the store and even more in a restaurant.

I try to keep a host of little serving-sized bags of pesto in the freezer that I make in the summer when I have lots of basil and other herbs in my garden or can get big bunches of it in the grocery store. I use walnuts if I can't afford the pine nuts and whip it up with olive oil, fresh garlic, and grated parmesan cheese. It's a shame to use it on store-bought pasta but we do it if we don't have the time or energy to make it.

This has been quite a long intro for such a short recipe. Oh well. Thinking about making your own pasta generally takes more time than actually doing it!

Take two eggs, some oil, and some flour. Add a pinch of salt if you like. Mix it up on your countertop until it's a good paste. Roll out as thinly as possible. I use a hand operated pasta press. Slice into noodles. Nothing is perfect, especially homemade stuff, just try to get them as even as possible. Let them dry out or cook them while still fresh. That's it. It takes less time to cook than commercial pasta.

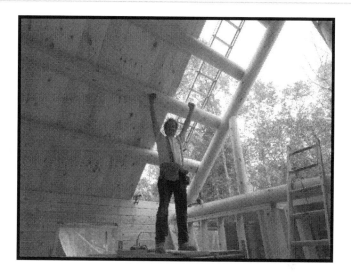

EPILOGUE
July 17, 2014

As I work steadily on helping Mike with house-building projects like stairs, closets, shelving, and other important jobs, I have begun writing Book II, and am reading through and organizing Book I to assure its quality and get it published. It is a full summer, a busy time of the year in every life. Last May, Mike and I cut our first tree to clear the property. We have worked steadily since then but are fully present and tireless in our work, as it contains authentic meaning for us and our family. We are fulfilling our dreams: our combined dream as a couple and our separate dreams as individuals.

Every night before bed, we pray for our friends, family and ourselves, that we may be guided to do only what serves goodness and light. We send a love bubble to our family members and know that they feel the embrace. We are here for them as a place of retreat or rest but, like so many people of our generation, cannot afford to support them financially. They must learn to be self-sufficient and to keep things simple too.

As a couple, our hope is that whatever we have experienced and learned may be of use to others, especially our offspring, as realistically, that is the best thing we can give them besides our undying love.

Each day Mike and I awaken with gratitude for each other, for those whom we love, and for the Great Creator who planted within us the seed of choice. We are grateful to our country, which, in spite of its ailments, is still a place where its people are free to realize their dreams.

We awaken each day to our own version of the American Dream and we work to keep it real. Integrity for us is key. If we say we are going to do it, we work hard until we do. Keeping things simple is vital because of that level of commitment. We have to be sure that we are doing it because it makes sense, not because it sounds cool or to try and make a point of some kind. This is just one couple's American Dream. Not a bad one, I might add, not too bad at all.

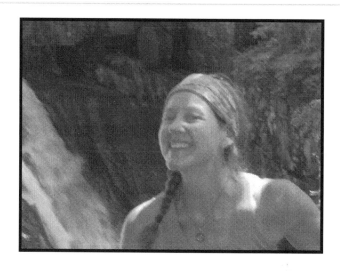

ABOUT THE AUTHOR

Michele Maingot Cabral spent her formative years climbing trees with pocket knives and notebooks. Her family consistently migrated between the United States and her father's homeland, Trinidad and Tobago. As a result of this transient childhood, she attended six elementary schools and happily learned to keep her own company. Her interest in writing continued into adulthood, as evidenced by boxes of journals and poetry that she shares sparingly.

Her main contribution to the human race has been the rearing of two loving daughters and a career as a high school English teacher. In that capacity, all writing awards were won by other people.

She now lives with her husband Mike and their dog Hermes in a partially-completed log cabin in the woods of Maine. She teaches writing, yoga, swings a hammer, keeps bees, gardens, and forages for a living. She and Mike also make a line of artisanal salves and soaps that they sell locally.

16310787R00098

Made in the USA
Middletown, DE
10 December 2014